Muscle Up

How Strength Training Beats Obesity, Cancer, and Heart Disease, and Why Everyone Should Do It

P. D. Mangan

Phalanx Press

Disclaimer: This book is for informational purposes only. The author is not a medical practitioner and the contents of this book do not constitute medical advice, which can only be given by a qualified medical practitioner. The information presented herein is believed to be accurate at the time of writing, but the author makes no warranties regarding its accuracy. The author and publisher shall not be liable for any omissions or inaccuracies or for any actions taken as a result of the contents of this book. The reader should consult a physician or other qualified medical professional before implementing any of the suggestions in this book and before beginning any exercise, diet, or fasting program and before taking any vitamin or other nutritional supplement. By purchasing this book, you agree to be bound by the terms of this disclaimer.

Table of Contents

Preface

What would you do if you discovered that all of the work you've been doing in the gym or exercising at home or outdoors was ineffective, or even worse, possibly destructive?

What if you found out that all of the exercise that you've spent years on was practically useless for either weight loss or for maintaining a normal body weight?

Would you be surprised to discover that all of the sweat and fatigue that you've put yourself through does little to slow many of the most important effects of aging?

I'm guessing that you would be annoyed if you discovered that much of what mainstream medicine has been telling you for decades is incomplete at best, and in some cases, even bad for your health. I know that I was annoyed when I figured it out.

The mainstream, both in medicine and in health and fitness circles, has told us for a long time now that everyone should do aerobic exercise, that it has unique powers to aid in weight loss, and that it's the only exercise you need to be healthy.

Wrong on both counts.

Aerobic exercise, which is what virtually everyone who exercises does, consists of activities like walking, jogging, and exercising on treadmills, stair steppers, and the like. In the gym it's often known as "cardio", for it's ability to raise the heart rate and improve cardiorespiratory fitness.

But despite what you may have heard, aerobic exercise has a terrible record at helping people lose weight. You may find that hard to believe, but I will scientifically document that statement in this book.

Aerobic exercise also does nothing to prevent the loss of muscle, and in some cases may even promote it, so it does nothing – or worse – to fight one of the biggest health problems of aging, muscle loss, which in its late stages is known as sarcopenia.

I won't go so far as to claim that aerobic exercise is bad for you – although in extreme cases, such as running marathons, it certainly can be. But if you're interested in your health, in losing fat or maintaining a normal body weight, and in feeling energetic, you can do much better.

Mainstream fitness started recommending aerobic exercise in a big way in the 1970s, at about the same time they began to recommend low-fat diets for health. It's now recognized that the low-fat diet era was a big mistake, that it may very well have inaugurated and sustained the obesity epidemic. Is it possible that the aerobic exercise era has also played a part in increasing the rate of obesity? Yes, it's certainly possible.

Aerobic exercise could have increased the rate of obesity in a couple of ways. One, by giving people the false idea that it can help weight loss through "burning" calories. Two, by unfounded claims that aerobic exercise is necessary and sufficient for good health, it discouraged people from taking up other forms of exercise that do have a better record at weight loss, mainly strength training.

Strictly aerobic exercise, the relatively low-level, steady-state kind exemplified by jogging, is not necessary for good health, since both strength training and high-intensity training improve cardiorespiratory fitness, as does aerobics.

Aerobic exercise is also not sufficient for good health, because it does little to nothing to increase whole-body muscle strength, a critical component of being healthy.

My aim in this book is to convince you that you should add strength training – also known as weightlifting or resistance training – to your exercise program. Hopefully you'll find that strength training, plus the occasional session of high-intensity training, is more than enough to keep you in excellent health with a highly fit body and you quit aerobics altogether.

It's a travesty that more people don't know about the health benefits of strength training. Mostly it's thought of as the province of a distinct and often derided class of exercisers, bodybuilders, who are (allegedly) interested in nothing more than big muscles, some of whom even take drugs to help them attain those muscles.

Strength training is not just for bodybuilders, however, it can and should be for almost everyone, whether they want bulging biceps and ripped abs or not. It can give energy and fitness to men and women and to the young, the middle-aged, and old, it can transform the fat, the skinny, and the weak, and it can restore the sick to health. It keeps body and mind in superb shape, and instills self-confidence and a sense of initiative.

In this book you'll see how strength training is the best exercise for fat loss, how it helps prevent cancer and heart disease, and fights the aging process. I'll discuss a related form of exercise, high-intensity training (HIT), and lastly you'll see how to implement a basic strength training program.

If you want to get better results from the time you spend on exercise, if you want to be healthier than plain old aerobic exercise can ever make you and to have a stronger and more attractive body than you've ever had, and to feel better than ever, this book, and strength training, are for you.

Chapter 1: Most people who exercise are not even trying

After many years in the gym I've noticed an odd but striking correlation – people who seem the most out-of-shape and in need of losing fat tend to do "cardio", or aerobics exercise. The correlation I've noted has not been subject to rigorous scientific study and has no p value (the scientific term for significance of results); it's just my own observation. But a person's apparent degree of fitness, as evidenced by his or her leanness and muscularity, seems to be inversely proportional to the amount of time he or she spends on treadmills, stair-steppers, and other cardio machines. Or maybe just outside walking or jogging for exercise.

By contrast, most of the really lean, muscular, and fit-looking people are lifting weights, whether using barbells and dumbbells or on machines.

Is this mere correlation or... could aerobic exercise and weightlifting each be causing the respective body types I associate with them? It's possible that it's just a coincidence: people who are overweight or otherwise out-of-shape find weightlifting too hard, or think that it is, and stick to aerobics. Muscular people, whether men or women, might find strength training more to their liking, perhaps easier than for the out-of-shape folks.

Besides the tentative fact that people with less muscle may find cardio easier and more to their taste than strength training, there's a widespread belief that cardio (aka aerobics or endurance exercise) is necessary for both fat loss and cardiovascular health. Unfortunately, ordinary aerobic exercise has quite a poor record when it comes to fat loss. The scientific record affirms this. And by ordinary aerobic exercise, I mean all those things that you normally see people do, whether in the gym or out, such as walking, jogging, or working out on aerobic exercise machines.

If you get to near marathon levels of aerobic exercise, you may be able to shed fat, but even there, marathon runners often have difficulty with weight gain.

As for cardiovascular fitness and health, aerobic exercise can indeed be helpful, but there are better ways to go about it, such as high-intensity training. Strength training itself also greatly improves cardiorespiratory fitness.

So maybe spending lots of time doing cardio *causes* a lack of fitness and leanness. That's to say, maybe cardio and aerobics are so ineffective for weight loss that those who practice this type of exercise remain overweight, or even become overweight despite it.

Steven Blair, a noted exercise scientist and himself a runner, wrote, "I often tell people that I was short, fat and bald when I started running, but that after running nearly every day for more than 30 years and covering about 70,000 miles...I am still short, fat, and bald. But I suspect I'm in much better shape than I'd be if I didn't run."[1] Yes, Blair may be fit in the cardiovascular sense, but after running 70,000 miles, he has lost little to no fat and for all we know probably gained some. Maybe if he had spent some of that time on strength training...well, he'd still be short and bald, but probably not so fat. It's remarkable that this idea doesn't even seem to have occurred to a scientist whose specialty is exercise. Such is the power of widely propagated ideas that many smart people don't even think to question them.

Heck, maybe cardio even *makes* people fat. That is not as outlandish an idea as it may sound.

Is there any evidence that strength training – also known as resistance training or weightlifting; it goes by many names, and I'm going to use these terms pretty much interchangeably – is better for fat loss than other types of exercise? As we shall see, yes, there is.

Why don't more people lift weights? Why do they spend so much time on treadmills, or walking, or other types of exercise that are relatively ineffective for fat and weight loss?

There are a number of reasons for this. One is that people have been told to do aerobic exercise for years now. Supposedly, you must have a so-called "aerobic" workout to improve your health and lose weight. While aerobic exercise isn't totally bereft of any health benefits, if your aim is to be efficient at getting in good cardiovascular condition and getting and staying lean, there are much better ways to exercise.

Mainstream fitness books and magazines have promoted the mistaken idea that getting out and walking thirty minutes a day is not only plenty of exercise, but that it will help you lose weight and maintain or attain good health. Now, don't get me wrong, I like and I do it myself on days when I'm not lifting weights. For someone who doesn't exercise at all, walking is a good place to start. For the elderly or infirm, walking might be the most they can manage, although even there, strength training works well and many of them are capable of it.

But you can do way better than walking or jogging or treadmills and stair-steppers.

Another reason more people don't do any kind of resistance training is that they perceive it as difficult and requiring special training. The weight room in the gym – and maybe even a few of the people in it – look unwelcoming to many, and that puts a few people off. All this, including the bit about unwelcoming weight rooms and some of the people in them, will be discussed later, but for now let's just say that those notions aren't completely reality-based.

Strength training is more intense than aerobic exercise

Strength training can seem difficult, especially at first and in comparison to aerobic exercise. It's more intense. If you're not used to it, picking up even a small dumbbell can feel like a challenge, and attempting bench presses or squats that exercise large muscle groups much more so.

In comparison, some of those cardio machines don't require a great deal of exertion. I've seen people reclining, reading the newspaper, and pushing pedals at a leisurely pace, and apparently they believe that this is exercise, though in reality it barely even qualifies.

I believe that both correlation and causation are at play in the relation between aerobics and not being in as good shape as one could: people find, or more likely, just think without trying it that weightlifting is too difficult, and therefore resign themselves to cardio, as a consequence of which they never get into very good shape; they never lose much fat, which, face it, is the reason most of them are in the gym. It's a vicious cycle: overweight → aerobics → no fat loss → more aerobics.

Strength training has been shown to have a dose-dependent relationship with change in waist size over several years, about twice as high as that for moderate to vigorous aerobic activity.[2] The connection between lower waist size and doing strength training could completely explain my observations concerning doing cardio and being out-of-shape and overweight. The authors of the study just cited conclude, "Substituting 20 min/day of weight training for any other discretionary activity had the strongest inverse association with WC [waist circumference] change… Among various activities, weight training had the strongest association with less WC increase."

The effect of weightlifting was far stronger for maintaining a lower waist circumference than for any other activity, in fact about twice as strong as for moderate to vigorous aerobic activity.

If you want to lose fat and/or stay lean, strength training is the way to do it. Get off the treadmill and hoist a few weights.

Waist circumference in turn is strongly correlated with percent body fat and insulin resistance, and is in fact a much better measure of body fat and health risk than the more traditional Body Mass Index (BMI). The reason for that is that a man (usually a man, but this can apply to women too) that has a lot of muscle mass can have a spuriously high BMI, since muscle is body weight also. But it's the amount, the percent, of body fat that burdens health. Extra muscle is in fact very healthy, because it burns more calories and greatly contributes to insulin sensitivity and thus better metabolism and a leaner physique.

Waist circumference also indicates the amount of abdominal or visceral fat, which is much more conducive to poor cardiovascular and metabolic health than subcutaneous fat. Abdominal fat is directly related to insulin resistance and the metabolic syndrome, which can lead to diabetes.

This suggests that strength training might be the best way to avoid metabolic illness, including diabetes, since this type of exercise is best for keeping your waist at a normal size.

For keeping your waist circumference in the normal, healthy range, weightlifting is your best bet.

Or, you could plod along on a treadmill for a few more years and see how that works.

You can't outrun a bad diet

Some people in my gym have been going at it on the cardio machines the entire time I've belonged to my gym, and their level of body fat doesn't appear to have changed at all. The lack of change is not merely due to the type of exercise that they do. It's also because you can't outrun a bad diet, and they don't know that.

People have been brainwashed into believing that exercise is as, or even much more, important for fat loss as is diet. It's easy to see why: both the fitness and food industries depend on it, so they fill their advertising with this idea. Most people get involved with the multi-billion dollar fitness industry – gym memberships, supplements, magazines and books, clothes and shoes – because they want to lose fat, and the fitness industry certainly doesn't want to disabuse anyone of the notion that their products and services will help people lose weight.

No, the fitness industry hides the fact that ordinary exercise has a poor record at weight loss because it wants to sell you its products. They promote the notion that their products and services will help people lose weight. Telling you that you need to cut down on or change what you eat doesn't sell many gym memberships, running shoes, or supplements.

On the other hand, the food and beverage industry doesn't want anyone to blame them for their overweight and obesity either. Profits depend on it. The food industry's blaming obesity on lack of exercise instead of their own products has been termed lean-washing.[3] In effect, the food and beverage industry says that *you* are the problem, because you're just too lazy or weak-willed to exercise enough. If only you would get off your lazy behind, they say, and exercise more, you could drink all the soda and eat all the pizza you want and stay lean. It's a blatant lie, but lies go around the world before the truth gets its boots on, and most people have accepted food biz propaganda without questioning it.

The fact is, the consensus of scientists and doctors who study and treat obesity, a consensus I agree with, is that diet is a far bigger determinant of body fat than is exercise. This comes with the important caveat that most of the forms of exercise that have been studied for weight loss have been traditional cardio-type exercises.

Aerobic exercise can increase your level of fitness, but without control of your diet, it will do almost nothing for weight loss. You may find it an exercise in futility.

Three doctors who are prominent in the study and treatment of obesity, Aseem Malhotra, Timothy Noakes, and Stephen Phinney, recently wrote an editorial for the *British Journal of Sports Medicine*: "It is time to bust the myth of physical inactivity and obesity: you cannot outrun a bad diet."[4] They note that science has shown little effect of exercise on weight loss, and state that many people still believe that obesity is a result of not enough exercise. In the opinion of these doctors, sugar in the diet has much more to do with obesity than lack of exercise. I agree. (Although other factors surely play a role, notably constant availability of food and around-the-clock eating.)

So all these people in my gym that have seen no change or become even fatter despite years of cardio may have been victims of the food and fitness industries' disinformation campaign and believe that they just need to aerobicize more. Or, of course, they don't know how to go about dieting. (Low-fat and low-calorie diets are not very effective, but that's a story for another time.)

Anyway, this isn't a diet book, but it bears stating that, to lose weight successfully, you need to get control of your diet. Resistance training can greatly help – avid bodybuilders eat mountains of food and still manage to maintain low body fat percentages. However, unless you're planning to go that route and lift heavy weights hard and daily, then some consideration of the type of food you eat will help fat loss on a resistance training program.

Strength training is a better solution to weight loss, but it must be done right

The correlation that I've observed between cardio and being out-of-shape isn't cut and dried, to be sure. Plenty of men – mostly men lift weights, although more women have been getting into it in recent years – haven't shown a lot of change in their body types either. That's because they're going about it the wrong way.

Too many people who lift weights focus on isolation exercises, that is, those exercises that revolve around one joint only and that isolate one muscle for exercise. Biceps curls and triceps pull-downs are examples of isolation exercise. While these exercises will help those isolated muscles to grow, they won't increase your cardiovascular fitness nor will they help you lose fat or really increase muscle overall.

In proper strength training, the best exercises are so-called compound exercises, which are those that revolve around two or more joints. Examples are bench or chest press, pull-downs or pull-ups, rows, squats, shoulder press, and deadlifts. These exercises will leave you breathing hard and with a fast heart rate, and in contrast to steady-state aerobic exercise, will actually lead to better body composition – more muscle and less fat. While more advanced strength trainers usually use free weights such as barbells and dumbbells to perform these, machines are perfectly fine. Machines might be the best choice for beginners and for older people, as they entail much less risk of injury, an important matter in resistance training.

In strength training, weights should be lifted with good form. Not doing so is a very common mistake.

Strength training necessarily requires a fair amount of exertion. Women – seems to be mostly women doing this – think they will get in shape by doing triceps extensions with a 5-pound dumbbell. Ain't gonna happen. If you're not grunting and groaning – or at least actively stifling your desire to do so – you're not training hard enough. This message was not approved by Planet Fitness.

I'm getting way ahead of myself. In the last chapter, we'll discuss all of this when we get to the basics of a strength-training program.

Sprint cycling and high-intensity training

There is one category of non-strength-training exercise in which I see some folks who are very much in shape, and that is the sprint cycling class. Now, this could be mere correlation too. It's a tough exercise regimen, so maybe only lean and fit people do it.

On the other hand, sprint cycling is not a form of steady-state aerobics – it's a form of high-intensity training (HIT), which has a much better basis both in theory and in practice for improving cardiovascular fitness and causing fat loss.

High-intensity training encompasses a great deal more than just sprint cycling. We'll discuss this type of exercise in more detail later, but keep in mind many or most of the health benefits of resistance training also apply to HIT.

My own story of strength training and health

Strength training played a key role in my journey from sickness to health. Aerobic exercise, specifically distance running, may have been important in my descent into ill health.

Back when I was around 20, running as exercise came into fashion and was promoted as a uniquely healthy exercise, so naturally I took up the sport, being the health-and-fitness-oriented guy that I am. Before too long, I was running greater distances and, eventually, I completed a couple of marathon races (26.2 miles).

My daily schedule always included running, usually somewhere between 4 and 8 miles daily, more on weekends.

Eventually, I came down with chronic fatigue, which has been shown to be more common among those who practice "extreme exercise". I don't want to place the entire blame for my illness on running, as I had a few other bad lifestyle habits that likely contributed to it, mainly being a vegetarian.

In any case, I was ill with chronic fatigue for many years, eleven to be precise. I saw many doctors and tried many things to try to overcome the illness.

One day when I was feeling a little bit better for whatever reason, I picked up a small barbell that I had laying around and worked out with it until I couldn't anymore, which was about 15 minutes.

And then I did it the next day, and then again a few days later. Before a month was out, I'd become stronger and realized I needed heavier weights, so I joined a gym.

I never looked back. I kept lifting weights and am still doing so many years later. My chronic fatigue is long gone, and I'm now 60 years old and in the best shape of my life. I feel fantastic and have energy to burn. I have under 12% body fat, and have no diabetes, heart disease, or any of that other crap that so many men my age have.

Now, I'm not saying that resistance training was the sole cause of my recovery from chronic fatigue, as I made a number of other changes, notably going on a low-carb high-fat paleo diet, as well as starting various dietary supplements. But weightlifting was a key element, and I feel sure I would not have recovered if not for that. (If you want to know more about how to recover from chronic fatigue, I wrote a book about it, ***Smash Chronic Fatigue***.)

Many years ago, on some now completely forgotten website, I read a brief remark by a young man who had some mysterious illness that none of his doctors could ever figure out. Eventually he went into a gym and started lifting weights, and he ultimately cured himself. Whatever his illness, whoever he was, I never forgot that, and ultimately I did the same. Young man, wherever you are, I salute you.

Strength training is a potent weapon in the fight against illness. I think you might be surprised at how much of your ill health it has the power to fix. This shouldn't be surprising, since muscle makes up a large portion of body mass, and it is highly involved in metabolism and health. If muscle tissue is tuned properly through strength training, and more muscle is added, better metabolic and cardiovascular health follows.

Exercise promotes health, but not all types of exercise are created equal

Exercise of all kinds promotes health and it's been said that if exercise were a pill, it would be the most widely prescribed one in the world. Unfortunately for the couch potatoes among us, it's not a pill and requires effort, which is why more people don't do it, and why doctors have all but given up trying to prescribe it. Face it, most people would rather take a pill, and doctors know this.

Some forms of exercise are far better than others for maintaining a healthy waist size or getting into good cardiovascular shape. Strength training and high-intensity training are much better for losing fat and attaining a lean muscular body.

As mentioned, diet is a necessary component of weight loss, despite what the fitness and food industries tell you. For fat loss, some of the most important muscles to exercise are the ones that push you away from the dining-room table. Although this book is about resistance training, most people get into the exercise game to lose fat, so for those of you like this, don't lose sight of the importance of a good diet, without sugar and low in refined carbohydrates like bread, pasta, and breakfast cereal, and with a healthy dose of protein.

Most people in the gym are not even trying. While I've emphasized here that strength training requires more effort, or more intense effort, than aerobic exercise, it can also be done in less time. Even as little as an hour a week can get you into better shape, with lower body fat, so in another sense it can be easier than aerobics.

If you want to get into the best shape ever, and perhaps most importantly, become healthier and reduce your risk of disease and death, try adding strength training to your exercise routine. In this book, I'll show you how and why it works, as well as introduce you to a basic strength training protocol.

Chapter 2: Weightlifting prevents cancer

No other intervention for health is as effective as exercise, and most people who exercise do it not just for the effect on weight loss, but because they want to improve their health. Yet some forms of exercise may be much better for health improvement than others. What would you think of a type of exercise that could keep you from getting cancer?

Cancer is one of the leading causes of death in the developed world. It is currently the second leading cause of death in the U.S., and is expected to surpass heart disease in the next few years to become the number one cause of death. Estimated new cases of cancer for 2015 come in at about 1.6 million, with deaths estimated at nearly 600,000.[5]

These are of course just the statistics. For a real person, a diagnosis of cancer is devastating; anxiety for the future, fear of death, and the prospect of a treatment nearly as bad as the disease loom large. It's safe to say that most people strongly fear the prospect of cancer, since the odds of it happening are real. One thing that makes this fear all the stronger is that, other than smoking, most people have no idea what causes cancer, and believe – mistakenly – that it just more or less strikes at random.

No, cancer does not strike at random. Obesity, for instance, is a major cancer risk factor.[6] Obesity could account for 14% of all cancer deaths in men, and 20% in women.[7] This data was from 2003, so the results are undoubtedly worse now and were probably an understatement to begin with. The American Cancer Society says that one out of every three cases of cancer are linked to either obesity, poor nutrition, or lack of physical activity.[8]

Physical fitness also has a strong inverse relation to dying from cancer.[9] The cited study states that "the risk of mortality from cancer declined sharply across increasing levels of fitness." Become fitter, and you have a far lower chance of getting cancer.

The fact is that one intervention greatly decreases the risk of cancer, and that is exercise, and even more so, resistance training. That's because not just fitness but muscular strength is associated with lower cancer risk.

The relationship between greater muscular strength and lower risk of cancer was discovered in a study that looked at people who enrolled at the Cooper Center in Dallas, Texas, which is known for its emphasis on aerobics, or endurance exercise.[10] The subjects studied were 8,677 men between the ages of 20 and 82, and followed from 1980 to 2003. The researchers quantified the men's muscular strength by their performance on bench press and leg press, their "1-repetition maximum" (1RM), which is the maximum amount of weight the subjects could move for one repetition.

The men were then grouped into thirds, "tertiles", according to strength, and then the researchers looked at how many of each group died of cancer. The group with the middle level of muscle strength had, when compared to the group with the lowest strength, a 35% reduced rate of cancer, and the group with the highest strength had a nearly 40% reduced cancer rate.

Now, it's known that levels of body fat, body mass index (BMI), waist circumference, and/or cardiorespiratory fitness are associated with cancer risk. The higher the numbers for the first three measures, and the lower for fitness, the greater the risk of cancer. But the study's authors found that after adjusting for muscular strength, the association of these risk factors with cancer disappeared.

In other words, muscular strength appeared to be the single most important factor of those measured for risk of getting cancer. Oddly, adjusting for cardiorespiratory fitness had little effect on the association. So at least some of the effect of muscle strength is due to exercise itself or to increased muscle mass.

Insulin-like Growth Factor 1

Weight training in certain modes can result in lower resting levels of insulin-like growth factor 1, or IGF-1, an important growth hormone.[11] IGF-1 has been implicated in the initiation and growth of cancer. This makes sense, since IGF-1 promotes tissue growth, and unrestrained growth of tissue is the hallmark of cancer. People who have a congenital deficiency of IGF-1, which is called Laron syndrome, have a virtually zero risk of cancer.[12] (Another effect of IGF-1 deficiency is that it results in very short stature.)

While humans need IGF-1 to have normal growth, after maturity it functions as a pro-aging factor.

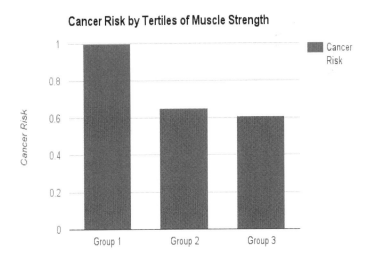

Cancer Risk by Tertiles of Muscle Strength

Centenarians typically have lower levels of IGF-1 than those who don't live that long.

The evidence linking IGF-1 to cancer is robust.[13] So, lowering IGF-1 may be an important way in which weightlifting can help prevent cancer. It may do this by increasing IGF-1 sensitivity.

However, the main reason that muscular strength reduces cancer may be because more muscle is associated with lower body fat, and body fat releases inflammatory chemicals ("cytokines"), and results in higher levels of insulin and IGF-1.

Bodybuilders typically want their levels of IGF-1 to increase, so there's something of a paradox here, since weightlifting can lower resting IGF-1, or at least does not increase it in the long term. But it appears that dietary protein is the main factor that raises IGF-1 levels. Not only that, but systemic IGF-1 does not appear to be important for building muscle; instead, weightlifting lowers levels of myostatin, which is the important driver of muscle growth or atrophy.[14]

To the extent that IGF-1 is necessary for muscle growth, it's IGF-1 that is produced in the muscle, and not systemically, that matters. IGF-1 in the circulation ("systemic IGF-1") is produced by the liver in response to dietary protein.

One thing to remember about cancer is that the risk of it greatly increases with age, so anything that retards the aging process necessarily has an anti-cancer effect. Strength training, and certain other exercise interventions, like high-intensity training (HIT), have the most potent anti-aging effects of any exercise.

Insulin is another hormone involved in aging and cancer. The beta cells of the pancreas release insulin in response to nutritional stimulus, mainly carbohydrates, and to a lesser extent protein. Insulin is of course necessary for life, but too much of it leads to illness, such as metabolic syndrome, diabetes, heart disease, and the topic of this chapter, cancer.

Scientists have linked excessive insulin to numerous types of cancer, including cancer of the breast[15], colon[16], ovaries, endometrial cancer, lymphoma, and leukemia.[17]

The good news is that strength training can radically increase insulin sensitivity, and thus decrease levels of insulin. Type 2 diabetics had a 48% increase in insulin sensitivity after just a few weeks of weight training.[18] One interesting point about this study is that the subjects were previously sedentary, and the exercise was characterized as being of "moderate" intensity. These people weren't bench-pressing 300 pounds or trying to become successful bodybuilders, but were simply working out in the gym, on machines, with 10 to 20 repetitions per exercise. Yet by laboratory evidence they became much healthier and lowered their risk of cancer.

Even the elderly can increase their insulin sensitivity and thus become healthier through weight training.[19]

One of the ways that resistance training increases insulin sensitivity is through increasing the number of glucose receptors, known as GLUT4, in trained muscle. These receptors bind to glucose in the bloodstream and take it up into the cells for use as fuel. In one study, diabetic patients increased the number of GLUT4 receptors by 40% after only 6 weeks of weight training.[20] Just think of how much better one can do with a concerted, long-term effort at weight training – you could possibly all but abolish insulin resistance. (This isn't to say that other factors aren't important in insulin sensitivity, such as the amount of refined carbohydrates you eat and whether you're lean or overweight – those factors are very important.)

While aerobic training can increase insulin sensitivity, the beauty of resistance training is that it works the entire musculature, and thus increases sensitivity in every muscle that's trained. The GLUT4 receptors are on the muscle cell surface, and for a muscle to have an increase of GLUT4, it must be trained. Aerobic training generally only works the legs and does not provide the robust muscular stimulus required on all the muscles of the body for better insulin sensitivity and lower insulin levels.

By lowering systemic levels of IGF-1 and insulin, and improving insulin sensitivity, weight training helps prevent cancer.

Myokines

Virtually all cells in the body release small proteins, called cytokines, that serve to communicate with other cells. Cytokines are important immune and inflammation signals. Recent research has found that muscle cells release their own types of cytokines, and these have been termed myokines.[21] Myokines are important to the effects of exercise on metabolism.

Exercise robustly effects immune function, and myokine signaling is probably important to this. Muscles produce myokines when contracting, that is, exercising. Strength training increases the release of myokines.

The hormone irisin is a myokine that has been investigated in recent years, and it has a strong anti-cancer effect.[22] The more muscle and less fat a person has, the more irisin they have.

What if you already have cancer, or are a cancer survivor?

For the unfortunate people who receive a diagnosis of cancer, rigorous treatment that often makes people ill and that's sometimes considered worse than the disease awaits. Cancer survivors often have a long haul in getting back to normal and returning to work.

The same research group that determined that greater muscular strength meant a greatly decreased risk of cancer also studied what happens when a group of cancer survivors undertake resistance training.[23] The level of resistance training was assessed by self-report; in other words, these people were not on any strict program, and many of them were very likely just casual gym goers who occasionally hoisted some iron.

The results are fairly startling: cancer survivors who participated in resistance training had a 33% lower risk of death from all causes, including cancer.

This one intervention, weight training, can mean a much greater chance at life for cancer survivors. Since about half of the people with cancer eventually die of their disease, you can see how powerful weightlifting is in this regard.

One research group wanted to see how a group of cancer survivors fared when they underwent "high-intensity physical training" and how it would affect their prospects of returning to work.[24] The exercise regimen consisted mainly of "high-intensity resistance training" supervised by an experienced physiotherapist. (The participants were also told to do endurance exercises such as walking and cycling at home, but this aspect was not supervised.) An age-matched control group received only "standard medical care". The exercise group returned to work two weeks sooner than the controls, were able to work more hours in the week, and in long-term follow-up, 78% of the strength training group had returned to work at the full number of hours they previously worked, versus 66% of the controls.

It must be concluded that resistance training is the best way to rehabilitate from cancer and from cancer treatment. Rest and standard medical care fared worse.

Some biomedical researchers believe that physical activity should be standard care in cancer treatment.[25] The beneficial effects of cancer therapy depend not only on the treatment itself, but on the general health of the patient, and exercise is one of the best ways to improve it. Quote: "Even though direct effects of physical activity on cancer are not definitively proven, given that physical activity is generally safe, improves quality of life for cancer patients, and has numerous other health benefits, *adequate physical activity should be a standard part of cancer care.*" [My emphasis].

The message: if you are a cancer survivor, better head to the gym. (Of course, run it by your doctor first.)

Cancer cachexia

Many patients who have cancer develop cachexia, which is a wasting condition in which they lose muscle and other lean tissue. Cachexia is caused by massive amounts of inflammation, either from the cancer or as a result of the treatment, and can be life-threatening.

One way in which cachexia is triggered is through increased levels of the hormone myostatin, which negatively regulates muscle growth. More myostatin means less muscle, and if myostatin can be lowered, then muscle can grow. In animal experiments, scientists found that increasing gene expression of myostatin prevented cancer cachexia.[26]

Weightlifting, as one might expect, decreases levels of myostatin, and this is one way in which this exercise causes muscles to grow. Weight training could be a solution for cachexia.

Patients with rheumatoid arthritis often develop cachexia, and so a trial of weightlifting was done on these patients with the object of seeing whether it would help muscle growth and reverse cachexia.[27] As with the study of cancer survivors, these "mildly disabled" people worked out relatively casually: an average 2.5 times a week for 10 weeks.

They gained an average of 1.2 kilograms (2.6 pounds) of muscle mass. The authors of the study concluded that resistance training is "an effective and safe intervention for stimulating muscle growth in patients with rheumatoid arthritis".

Experiments have shown that animals that overexpress a certain molecule called PGC-1α "show increased muscle mass and strength and *dramatic resistance to the muscle wasting of cancer cachexia*."[28]

And how does one increase levels of PGC-1α? "Expression of PGC-1α4 is preferentially induced in mouse and human muscle during *resistance exercise*." Ergo, resistance training fights cancer cachexia.

A meta-analysis (a review of previously published scientific studies) took a look at what happened to cancer survivors doing resistance training.[29] While the study did not look at mortality rates, it did find "clinically important" effects, mainly an increase in muscle mass, which is important to those who have had cancer.

It's well known that weight loss during cancer and cancer treatment is a big problem, and that goes especially for loss of muscle. Resistance training can help add muscle. Of course whether any given cancer patient will be able to undergo this kind of training will greatly depend on an individual's circumstances, type of cancer, general health, and so on.

Less myostatin means longer life

We noted above the importance of myostatin in cancer cachexia. In patients with cancer, myostatin increases even before cachexia is evident.

Also as noted, aging greatly increases the risk of cancer, so anything that can slow or reverse the aging process can decrease the risk of cancer. One candidate molecule the decrease of which may counteract aging is myostatin, which is a myokine that inhibits muscle growth and differentiation.

It's been found that animals, in this case mice, that have been genetically engineered to have lower levels of myostatin, live much longer, as much as 15% longer, than regular ("wild type") mice.[30] More myostatin increases sarcopenia, or muscle wasting, and this seems to be intimately connected to lifespan. (We'll discuss sarcopenia more extensively in another chapter.) Myostatin is interesting as an apparent case in which growth, muscle growth in this case, results in greater longevity. Scientists haven't ironed out all the wrinkles in that idea yet.

Weightlifting robustly decreases levels of myostatin.[31] Therefore resistance training is a great place to start your anti-cancer and anti-aging program.

Takeaway Points

- Cancer will soon overtake heart disease as the leading cause of death in the U.S.
- Cancer does not strike randomly, but is associated with, among other things, obesity and lack of physical fitness.
- Greater muscular strength is strongly associated with lower risk of cancer.
- Strength training with weights or machines increases muscular strength.
- Strength training results in lower death rates in cancer survivors.
- Strength training improves insulin sensitivity.
- Strength training fights cachexia.
- Strength training lowers levels of myostatin, and thus combats aging.

Chapter 3: Weightlifting prevents cardiovascular disease

Cardiovascular disease is the leading cause of death

Heart disease is currently the leading cause of death in the U.S, for both men and women.[32] About 610,000 people die annually of heart disease, and every year about 750,000 people have a heart attack.

Each year nearly 800,000 Americans have a stroke, and strokes kill about 130,000 people annually[33], making it the number five cause of death.

Both coronary heart disease and stroke are cardiovascular diseases, often abbreviated CVD.

Both of these diseases occur when a blood clot or piece of broken arterial plaque blocks an artery, causing death of tissue when the blood supply is cut off, either in the heart or in the brain. A number of conditions raise the risk of CVD, including high blood pressure, smoking, obesity, sedentary lifestyle, insulin resistance, and diabetes.

Exercise is known to be a major preventative of CVD. What we want to look at here of course is whether there's any special case to be made for resistance training in the prevention of CVD.

Greater muscle strength means less cardiovascular disease

Grip strength is a simple, easy-to-use measurement of muscle strength. So what happens when you measure grip strength and then follow the subjects for many years after?

A study undertaken in Japan did just that.[34] The study had nearly 5,000 subjects, a number that should be large enough to give reasonable, statistically significant answers. It included both men and women.

It found that men who were in the highest fifth (quintile) of muscle strength had a risk of death that, depending on age, was from about one third to one half lower than those in the middle fifth. Specifically regarding CVD, each 5 kilogram increment in grip strength meant a 15% (for heart disease) or 10% (for stroke) lower risk of death. The results were similar in women.

In a survey done in the UK, nearly 200,000 people, aged 65 and older, had their grip strength measured, and were then followed for several years after.[35] For men, each one standard deviation (SD, a statistical measure) increase in grip strength meant a 27% lower risk of cardiovascular death.

At a one SD increase in grip strength, you'd be in about the top one third of all people in terms of strength, and would have a CVD risk only 73% that of those with average grip strength. At a two SD increase in strength, you would be in the top 5%, and would have a risk of CVD only about half that of those in the middle. Of course your risk would be way lower than those with below-average strength.

With a regular strength training program, you could easily put yourself into the top one third of people who are the same age, and probably even into the top 5%, and thus dramatically lower your risk of heart disease and stroke. If that seems unlikely, consider that probably 99% of all people do no strength training, so if you're, say, a 70-year-old who does train for strength, you'll readily outclass almost everyone else, even if you don't train all that hard.

The chart below shows the survival curves for the men and women who were measured according to thirds of grip strength. (This shows deaths from all causes, not just CVD.) Recall that when grip strength was measured, all the subjects were 65 or older – just so you won't be too startled at seeing how quickly after the measurement people started dying.

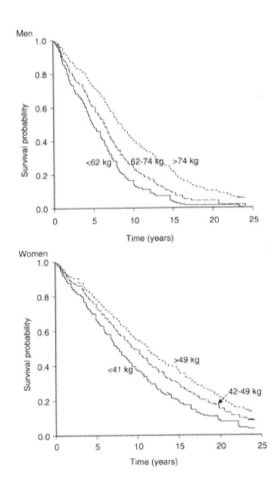

In ten years time, those with high grip strength were approximately 50% more likely to be alive, and in 15 years, the chance was about 100% greater.

These results show that muscular strength is an important predictor of mortality, including CVD mortality.

The authors of this study suggest that "that the influence of grip strength on survival may have more to do with the effectiveness with which muscle functions than its size." They also note that poor grip strength is associated with insulin resistance, which precedes diabetes and is highly involved in promoting heart disease. (One school of thought, one I'm inclined to agree with, holds that insulin resistance is the major cause of heart disease, of which more below.)

Does that mean that increasing muscular strength through weight training will decrease your risk of heart disease? The short answer is yes; the longer answer, also yes, is that increasing muscular strength means better insulin sensitivity, and thus a lower rate of all the diseases caused by it, including heart disease, cancer, diabetes, and obesity.

Besides muscular strength, strength training also favorably affects CVD risk markers, such as blood pressure, fat mass, and triglyceride levels.[36]

Muscle mass is an important determinant of CVD risk, and lower muscle mass, whether through aging, being sedentary, hospitalization, or a poor diet, can lead to obesity, diabetes, and hypertension, all of which increase the risk of CVD.[37] Strength training increases muscle mass, and as such lowers that risk. Muscle mass is by weight the largest tissue in the body and has an important role in metabolism, taking up glucose and fats from the circulation.

Men with greater muscular strength, in the highest third as measured by bench and leg presses, had a 30% lower risk of dying from CVD than those in the bottom third.[38] So it's not just some fluke of grip strength that predicts mortality—it's *total body strength*.

Total aerobic fitness is an important concept in cardiovascular disease, since the better your aerobic fitness, the less likely you are to get heart disease or stroke. Aerobic fitness is usually measured by VO_2max, which is the rate at which a person can maximally take up oxygen. Exercise training increases this measure, that is, if the exercise is hard enough. (For example, walking will not usually improve oxygen uptake, unless one is in poor shape to begin with.) Strength training significantly improves VO_2max.[39] This is important to note because of a common belief that only aerobic training, or "cardio", has the capacity to improve VO_2max.

The fact is, if lifting is done properly, your heart and respiratory rates will become substantially elevated, which shows that it is indeed hard exercise for the circulatory system. Does one need to do "aerobics" in addition to weightlifting? It may be helpful for attaining peak cardiovascular fitness, although as we'll see in another chapter, high-intensity training is better, but if you do nothing but regular resistance training, your fitness and risk markers will greatly improve.

As an illustration, let's see what happens when men aged 60 to 75 go through a program of high-intensity resistance training. In this form of strength training, participants push themselves very hard. They did 3 sets of each exercise at 6 to 8 repetitions per set, to failure, meaning that they used weights such that 6 to 8 reps was the most they could do before they could do no more ("failure"). The program lasted 16 weeks. Another group of men did not train and served as the control group.[40]

The men's body fat dropped by 3 percentage points, strength went way up, and VO_2max and treadmill performance increased. They greatly improved in matters of cardiorespiratory fitness, exactly where you want to see improvement in order to prevent cardiovascular disease.

While the program that these older men went through may seem a tough one, the authors of this study commented, "Older men may not only tolerate very high intensity work loads but will exhibit intramuscular, cardiovascular, and metabolic changes similar to younger subjects."

I imagine that the first reaction of many older people to the idea of resistance training is that it's too difficult, and that they're too old for it. This study shows that nothing could be further from the truth.

Another study looked at the outcome of a 6-month resistance training program in men and women aged 60 to 83.[41] The subjects again increased their strength, aerobic capacity went up, and treadmill time increased by about 25%, a solid gain in aerobic fitness.

What if you already have cardiovascular disease?

If you already have some form of cardiovascular disease, the same caveats apply to resistance training as they do to other forms of exercise. The amount and type of exercise that you do depends on factors like your age, your previous level of fitness, and perhaps most importantly, the severity of the underlying cardiovascular disease that you have. Your doctor also needs to sign off on any exercise program you might undertake.

The American Heart Association Council on Clinical Cardiology and Council on Nutrition, Physical Activity, and Metabolism issued an extensive, joint scientific statement on the rationale and benefits of resistance training in individuals with regard to CVD: "Resistance Exercise in Individuals With and Without Cardiovascular Disease".[42] They state:

"... RT [resistance training] has become even more accepted and commonly used in exercise training programs for persons with and without CVD. The potential benefits, not only to cardiovascular health but also to weight management and the prevention of disability and falls, are becoming more widely appreciated. For persons at low risk for cardiac events, extensive cardiovascular screening is probably not necessary, although a graded approach is recommended. For persons at moderate to high risk of such events, RT can be safely undertaken with proper preparation, guidance, and surveillance.... However, given the extensive evidence of the benefits of aerobic exercise training on the modulation of cardiovascular risk factors, RT should be viewed as a complement to rather than a replacement for aerobic exercise."

As you can see, the AHA wants you to do aerobic exercise in addition to resistance training. It's my belief that high-intensity training makes a better complement to strength training, but be that as it may, strength training alone also improves cardiovascular fitness, at least when done in the right way.

Takeaway Points

- Cardiovascular disease is the leading cause of death
- Greater muscle strength is associated with less CVD and lower death rates
- Strength training increases cardiorespiratory fitness
- If you already have CVD, strength training can help

Chapter 4: Weight training keeps you lean and improves metabolic health

Many people who exercise do so because it helps them, or they believe that it helps them, lose weight. Sure, plenty of people are in the gym – or out walking or running – for the health benefits. Some are even there to socialize, especially in fitness classes. But with the obesity epidemic making two out of every three Americans overweight (Body Mass Index, or BMI, ≥ 25) or obese (BMI ≥ 30), and judging by who goes to the gym, I think it's safe to say that losing weight—specifically, fat – or maintaining a healthy body weight motivates large numbers of people.

The problem there is that ordinary exercise has a poor record at promoting weight loss, as we saw in the first chapter of this book.

Why is that exactly? The fitness industry and media constantly promotes the idea of "burning" calories through exercise, and most people who exercise buy into this idea. But there are a few obvious difficulties with it.

For one thing, exercise doesn't really burn all that many calories. For instance, walking burns about 100 calories a mile, so if you walked at a decent clip, you'd burn 400 calories in an hour. Or say that you run; running burns about the same number of calories per mile, so if you run 4 miles, it will take less time than walking, but burn approximately the same number of calories. Many people never even get to this level; most walkers and runners are not doing 4 daily miles. And by the way, those figures for calories burned include your basal metabolic rate, which is around 80 calories an hour when awake. In other words, those 400 calories you "burned" while out walking is only 320 more than you would have burned sitting on the sofa at home.

It's extremely easy to eat enough to make up for that. A typical fast-food meal, a burger, fries, and a drink, may have 1000 calories or more. A few cookies alone may make up for those 400 calories you just "burned off". White Russian at your favorite bar? 300 calories. White chocolate mocha at Starbucks? 620 calories. Add to that the fact that so many people "reward" themselves with something tasty after a bout of exercise, and you can see why the idea of "burning" calories with exercise is only just short of nonsense.

The main problem with using exercise to burn calories or lose fat is that exercise makes you hungry, and if you're hungry, sooner or later you're going to eat, and it's very easy to make up for, or even exceed, the amount of calories you've burned.

Cases abound of people, even elite athletes, who gain weight while burning thousands of calories in daily exercise. Consider the case of Peter Attia, a physician and now one of the leading lights behind NuSI, the Nutrition Science Initiative, whose goal is to settle once and for all some of the main scientific problems in the field of nutrition. A competitive swimmer, Attia wrote, "Despite exercising 3-4 hours per day, I had morphed from a lean person into a sort of chubby guy over the preceding several years. In high school I weighed 160 pounds and carried about 5-6% body fat (9 pounds of fat on my body). I had ballooned to as high as 200 pounds with 25% body fat (50 pounds of fat on my body)." This is a man who has swum the Catalina Channel.

Attia, like most people, was under the delusion that lots of exercise kept fat off, and that you didn't really need to watch what you eat when burning calories at such a prodigious rate. "I exercised more in one day than the average person did in one week. I didn't eat at McDonalds or Taco Bell."

Attia eventually lost 25 pounds of pure fat by eliminating sugar from his diet and keeping his carbohydrate intake to around 50 grams a day.[43]

Marathon runners can also put on lots of fat tissue, believe it or not. So-called experts have recommended that distance runners eat lots of carbohydrates, and if they follow this prescription faithfully, can gain a lot of weight. The weight isn't muscle either, it's fat. A recent article in the Boston *Globe* states, "Marathon-training-induced weight gain is so prevalent that it's been studied by researchers and addressed by Runner's World magazine, which periodically runs stories with headlines that read as if plucked from the satirical Onion publication: "How to Avoid Marathon-Training Weight Gain," and "10 Tips to Avoid Weight Gain While Training."" As usual, runners think that they're burning off so many calories that they don't need to watch what they eat.

Of course, people who have trouble with gaining fat even in the face of lots of exercise are often doing the wrong kind of exercise. Marathon runners often look positively sickly due to the loss of large amounts of muscle. Aerobic exercise doesn't build muscle, which is an essential component of any exercise that will help you lose weight. Strength training helps you to keep or in most cases even build more muscle.

Most people who attempt to lose weight do so not through exercise alone but through a combination of diet and exercise. However, one thing that almost inevitably happens when anyone loses weight is that, in addition to losing fat, they lose muscle, which is an unhealthy situation that makes it more difficult to lose fat, and also encourages weight regain since it decreases the metabolic rate, i.e. the body burns less energy.

Muscle burns calories at a much higher rate than fat tissue, so the more muscle and less fat that a person has, the higher their metabolic rate will be, which means simply that your thermostat is set a bit higher and you burn more energy.

How much more energy does muscle burn? This has been disputed, since resting muscle doesn't require all that many calories. What is missed in the dispute, however, is that muscle turns over, that is, it breaks down and builds up daily, and this requires energy.

Muscle burns enough energy that at the extremes, for example comparing a young, well-muscled man to an elderly woman, the difference in resting energy expenditure could be as much as 365 calories a day.[44] If other things are equal, such as calorie intake, then this leads to a gain or loss of about 1.4 kg (~3.1 pounds) of fat a month. Which is huge. Even a mere 100 calorie a day difference in energy expenditure can mean 4.7 kg (over 10 pounds) difference in fat weight a year.

If you've wondered why, as you get older, eating the same amount of food that kept you lean and trim when you were young now causes you to get fat, the answer is because when you were young you had a lot more muscle. (And this applies to both men and women.) All that muscle of youth means that the young burn calories at a much higher rate, even with no exercise. The melting away of muscle with age decreases the basal metabolic rate, so if you don't decrease the number of calories you ingest, boom, you get fat.

Instead of trying to burn calories through walking on a treadmill, put on some muscle so that you burn extra calories around the clock, not just when exercising. Resting muscle preferentially burns fat too.

Strength training prevents muscle loss when dieting

You hardly ever hear this in discussion of diet and weight loss, but low-calorie diets don't just cause the loss of fat, but of muscle as well. A rule of thumb has it that for every four pounds of fat you lose, you will also lose one pound of muscle. Ideally, you want to lose no muscle at all, just fat. Losing muscle is bad for health and for weight maintenance.

In a study that demonstrated how dieters lose muscle along with fat, researchers put a group of people on a very low calorie diet, 800 calories a day, and the subjects stayed on this for twelve weeks. One part of the group was put on the diet plus aerobic exercise, and the other went on the diet, but did resistance training three times a week instead.[45] One guess as to what happened.

As you might expect, both groups lost a significant amount of weight. The diet plus aerobics group lost 18 kilograms (almost 40 pounds), compared to a loss of 14.4 kg (about 32 pounds) for the diet plus resistance training group. Unfortunately, about 4 kg (almost 9 pounds) of the weight loss in the aerobics group was lean mass, which is to say, muscle. The resistance training group lost 14.4 kg, *all of which was fat.* They lost no muscle.

The 9 lost pounds of muscle in the diet plus aerobics group results in worse health, and likely represents muscle that they will never get back. The diet plus strength training group undoubtedly improved their health, since their weight loss was pure fat.

In the aerobics group, the resting metabolic rate as a function of lean mass decreased, while it increased in the resistance training group.

Furthermore, VO_2max, the most important measure of cardiorespiratory fitness, increased to the same extent in both groups, another demonstration that resistance training is as effective as aerobics in this regard.

Another study, perhaps more realistic in that that the diet was 80% of normal daily intake, looked at the effect of dieting plus strength training plus extra protein on loss of fat and muscle.[46] The subjects were all overweight policemen.

The subjects, all of them men, were placed into three groups:

- diet only
- diet + resistance training + 70 grams casein protein supplement daily
- diet + resistance training + 70 grams whey protein supplement daily

The extra protein in the supplemented groups brought their protein intake up to 1.5 grams of protein per kilogram of body weight daily, or about 25%

of total calories.

The resistance training program consisted of 30 minutes of training on 4 days a week; it was performed on exercise machines and was supervised by an experienced physical trainer.

The diet alone group lost 2.5 kg (5.5 pounds) of fat, with an insignificant loss of lean mass, which probably occurred because the diet was not that low in calories, and the amount of total weight loss was low. Still, a mere 5.5 pounds fat loss seems like little to show for 12 weeks of low-calorie dieting. That's less than one pound a week, and if you needed to lose a substantial amount of weight, would take quite awhile.

In contrast, the group that dieted and performed resistance training and took extra protein in the form of casein lost about 7 kg (15 pounds) of fat, and gained 4 kg (9 pounds) of lean mass, that is, muscle. The whey group lost 4.2 kg (9 pounds) of fat, and gained 2 kg (4.4 pounds) of lean mass.

With resistance exercise and extra protein, it is possible to maintain and even gain lean mass while losing weight. The diet alone group lost a small amount of lean mass, although the study considered the amount insignificant.

These results lay to rest the bodybuilding myth that it's difficult to gain muscle and lose fat at the same time. These dieters gained muscle – a lot of it. Granted, they were beginning strength trainers and overweight, and if you're already decently fit with relatively low body fat, it's going to be more difficult. That's just how it is: dialing down body fat from low levels to very low levels, as bodybuilders often do, is tough. But if you're trying simultaneously to lose fat and build muscle starting at the level most people start from, it certainly is possible. Given how many Americans are in the same kind of condition as the policemen in the study – very overweight and out-of-shape – many people, I would say most, should be capable of this.

The point for anyone trying to lose weight through dieting is that adding resistance training to your weight loss efforts is very beneficial, both for your weight loss and for your health. You can add muscle, and keep your metabolic rate – the amount of calories you burn at rest – high. Maintaining a decently high metabolic rate is important in weight loss, since when people lose weight, typically their metabolic rate declines, and then they have difficulty losing more weight, or even begin to regain it. There's also the matter of how one feels; generally, the higher your metabolic rate, the more energy you will have and the better you feel.

Strength training prevents muscle loss when on a low-calorie diet, and in many cases it can even add muscle while dieting. Aerobic exercise on a low-calorie diet can lead to loss of muscle, potentially worsening health and sabotaging healthy weight maintenance.

The choice of exercise for weight loss is clear. Strength training beats aerobic exercise hands down.

Resistance training and waist circumference: body composition is paramount for health

In the first chapter, I mentioned the results of a study that looked at the relation between waist circumference and weightlifting.[47] The study found that weightlifting was far more effective at keeping increasing waist size at bay than aerobic activity. Specifically, each 20-minute daily increment of weight training was associated with 2/3 centimeter smaller waist size.

If you have a normal body weight, why should you care about waist circumference? Other than for appearance, that is: most people intuitively understand and want a lower waist size.

Normally we are accustomed to seeing Body Mass Index (BMI) as a measure of normal, overweight, or obese body types. BMI has a big drawback, however, namely that it doesn't distinguish between fat and muscle. Only excess fat is deleterious for health; extra muscle is better for health. A man or woman who has a lot of extra muscle can register as overweight or obese when BMI is used as a measurement, but in reality they're at a perfectly healthy weight. This situation doesn't arise that often, however, since so few people have enough extra muscle to increase their BMI much, so health researchers looking at population-level statistics can effectively ignore it. That's one reason that they continue to use BMI as a measure of health risk. If everyone took up strength training and added muscle, health scientists would need to adjust the BMI numbers upward as a measure of overweight and obesity.

BMI is meant to measure excess fat. Measuring the amount of body fat directly is a much better measure of health risks. So why isn't percent body fat used more often?

While percent body fat is a more accurate measure of the impact of weight on health, it requires specialized equipment to measure properly, such as the instrumentation used for a DEXA scan, and this costs more, requiring a trained technician, specialized equipment, and time to do so, i.e. an appointment; it's not offered everywhere, certainly not in a typical doctor's office, and not even in most gyms.

Waist size, on the other hand, requires only a tape measure. The difference in the amount of health risk between waist circumference and BMI can be startling.

To give an idea of the difference between BMI and waist circumference as they impact health, take a look at the following chart.

The chart shows the prevalence of various diseases, including metabolic syndrome, diabetes, hypertension, and cardiovascular disease, in people with a *normal BMI*, but grouped by tertiles (thirds) of waist size. Technically, with a normal BMI, these people are not even overweight. Their doctors would look at their BMI and tell them that they're fine.

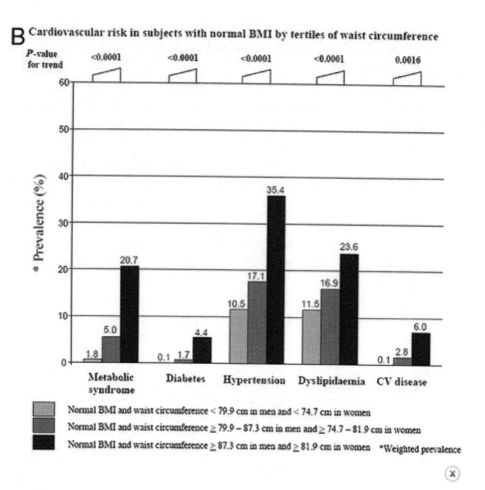

B Cardiovascular risk in subjects with normal BMI by tertiles of waist circumference

Normal BMI and waist circumference < 79.9 cm in men and < 74.7 cm in women

Normal BMI and waist circumference ≥ 79.9 – 87.3 cm in men and ≥ 74.7 – 81.9 cm in women

Normal BMI and waist circumference ≥ 87.3 cm in men and ≥ 81.9 cm in women   *Weighted prevalence

Only the people with low waist circumference are fine, however. *Within the normal weight category*, men with a waist circumference greater than 87.3 cm (34.4 inches), and women with a waist larger than 81.9 cm (32.2 inches) *had 11.5 times the rate of metabolic syndrome, 44 times the rate of diabetes, and a whopping 60-fold increase in the rate of cardiovascular disease.*[48]

This condition, a normal BMI with a high waist circumference, is known as "normal weight obesity", and it is a risk factor for the metabolic syndrome – leading to type 2 diabetes – and death from cardiovascular disease. In normal weight obesity, body weight is technically within a normal range, as indicated by Body Mass Index, but too little muscle and too much fat combine to make this condition every bit as risky for health as regular obesity.

In other words, just because you have a normal BMI, it doesn't mean that you're out of the woods health wise.

Body composition, that is, the relative amounts of muscle and fat, is paramount for health, not BMI or absolute weight. Fat mass, not body weight, increases health risks. *The only exercise regimen that will help improve and maintain a body composition favorable for health is resistance training.* This can be seen in the above cited studies showing that weightlifting keeps waist circumference low, and that higher waist circumference is associated with much higher risk of disease and death.

If someone tries to lose weight using conventional diet and aerobic exercise, they run the risk of loss of lean body mass and placing themselves into the "normal weight obese" category and increasing their risk of serious illness.

Any attempt at weight loss should always be accompanied by strength training of some kind in order to avoid loss of lean muscle mass.

Greater muscular strength means lower risk of obesity

A person who has greater muscular strength is also less likely to be obese in the first place.[49] Men who are in the highest quintile (fifth) of muscular strength have sharply lower odds of obesity compared to those in the lowest, as much as 70% lower. To avoid obesity, one should increase and/or maintain a healthy level of muscle mass.

The authors of the cited study that found that strength protects against obesity speculated on why that should be, and noted that in experimental animals, muscle hypertrophy (growth) resulted in "reductions in body weight, fat mass, plasma glucose, insulin, and leptin." These measurements are all important in good metabolic control, i.e. lower risk of diabetes and heart disease. They also noted that "when the muscular hypertrophy was experimentally blocked, the positive effects were completely abolished."

They conclude that "interventions to produce muscular hypertrophy... may prove to be critical weapons in the fight against obesity and obesity-related comorbidities [illnesses]."

The most robust intervention that produces muscular hypertrophy is resistance training.

Muscle is a highly metabolically active tissue, and it competes for and takes up glucose and fats for the nutrients it needs for energy and growth. Increasing the amount of muscle mass leads to more nutrients shuttled to the muscle rather than other tissues, particularly fat. When muscle metabolizes and grows, fewer nutrients are available for the growth of fat tissue. This is one of the explanations for more muscle leading to less fat.

The growth of fat tissue requires the presence of the hormone insulin, which is produced by the pancreas and is strongly stimulated by dietary carbohydrates. Strength training produces a robust increase in insulin sensitivity, so that the body requires less insulin for the necessary regulation of glucose and other nutrients. Insulin levels drop and as a consequence, abundant insulin is no longer pushing nutrients into fat tissue for storage. Lower insulin levels also allow fat to leave fat tissue, leading to fat loss.

A recent report found that losing weight can actually be dangerous to your health.[50] People with a higher BMI had a lower risk of death. But just as we saw above, higher waist circumference was associated with a higher risk of death. It's all about the relative amounts of body fat and muscle.

Losing weight can be bad for health if not done properly, which is by minimizing muscle loss. Losing abdominal and subcutaneous fat is the healthy aspect of weight loss. (Other measures besides resistance training, such as decreasing the intake of refined carbohydrates and increasing protein intake, also cause a shift in weight loss away from muscle and toward fat tissue.)

Does aerobic exercise actually make you fat?

Well, that's a provocative statement, isn't it? It goes against everything that has ever been said about exercise and body weight. But there's evidence to at least suggest that aerobic exercise could make people fat.

Take the example of walking, the most common and most recommended aerobic exercise. If a person's sole exercise is walking, he or she stands to lose 4 to 6 pounds of muscle and reduce their metabolic rate by 2 to 3% per decade, which is no different from no exercise at all.[51] If that loss rate for muscle tissue and metabolism goes on for decades, you have a recipe for sarcopenia, low metabolism leading to obesity, and just all around feeling lousy, with no zest for life. All of this could happen even if you religiously follow your doctor's and mainstream medicine's advice to walk for exercise.

But consider that in 10 weeks of resistance training, only 2 days a week, a group of people, ages 20 to 82, lost nearly 2% of their body fat and gained 3 pounds of muscle. This was undoubtedly a better result than if they had spent decades walking.

Walking is the most commonly prescribed form of exercise, and is what doctors recommend most often to their patients. *Yet in terms of muscle loss, walking is no better than no exercise at all.* Since losing muscle sets a person up for fat gain, doing nothing but walking could, in the long term, lead to becoming overweight. Q.E.D.: aerobic exercise can make you fat.

48

Many people who do aerobic exercise "reward" themselves for having exercised, and as we noted, they're hungrier too, and they tend to eat highly refined carbohydrates, which they've been told is the right fuel for this particular type of activity. Result: fat gain.

Aerobic or endurance exercise, especially of a long duration, also causes an increase in the hormone cortisol, and this not only leads to fat storage, but loss of muscle, since cortisol is a catabolic hormone, meaning that it breaks down lean tissue.

In men, endurance training can lead to a hypogonadal state, with low testosterone levels[52], which is another way that aerobic exercise can lead to loss of lean mass and fat gain, not to mention the crimp it can put in a man's sex life.

Strength training, in contrast, *increases* testosterone in men.

So aerobic exercise can potentially make people fat in several ways:

- by failing to prevent muscle loss, leading to poor metabolism
- by increasing cortisol, which can *cause* muscle loss
- by giving people an excuse to reward themselves with food
- by decreasing testosterone in men, leading to less muscle and more fat tissue.

The solution is to skip the aerobics and strength train instead.

Metabolic health

Insulin and insulin resistance has been strongly implicated in the development of obesity and the inability to lose weight. We've already covered some of the mechanisms behind the ability of strength training to reduce insulin levels and increase insulin sensitivity. This arguably has much to do with the better record of resistance training when it comes to fat loss.

Much of the increased insulin resistance in the obese and the elderly is due to the increased fat mass that seems to magically appear with age, and resistance training can greatly assist in preventing both the fat and the insulin resistance. Some of the increased insulin resistance seen in these people may also be caused by changes in the muscle itself, specifically its inability to metabolize fats properly. In this model of insulin resistance, exercising muscle through strength training can restore proper metabolism to muscle, thus preventing insulin resistance and the obesity and diabetes that accompany it.

So, strength training, in contrast to aerobic exercise, fights insulin resistance in both of these ways: keeping fat low and maintaining or increasing muscle mass, and by improving muscle function and metabolism.

In just a few short weeks, strength training can improve insulin sensitivity much more than if you did aerobic exercise for the same length of time.

Takeaway points

- Ordinary (aerobic) exercise has a poor record at weight loss
- Weight loss is often accompanied by muscle loss
- You can be obese even at a normal weight if muscle mass is low
- Waist circumference measures body fat better than Body Mass Index (BMI)
- Resistance training is about twice as effective as aerobic exercise in decreasing waist circumference
- Greater muscular strength means lower risk of obesity

- Any weight loss attempt should be accompanied by resistance training

Chapter 5: Strength training fights aging

Aging means an increase in the incidence and likelihood of becoming ill and a decrease in the body's capacity for self-renewal. When we're younger, the body renews itself and repairs damage much more readily than when we get older. Aging is often thought of as "falling apart", and that expression contains more than a grain of truth.

Exercise remains one of the most potent prescriptions for fighting aging. People who exercise have much lower rates of illness such as cancer and heart disease, and a much lower chance of dying in any given time period – a lower mortality rate, to use the jargon.

Steady-state aerobic exercise, the kind that has long been recommended and the type almost everyone does, improves health but has a number of disadvantages when it comes to aging. One main disadvantage is that it does little to prevent the gradual breakdown of tissues seen in aging, and in fact may even accelerate it by causing muscle loss.

Anyone serious about slowing or reversing the aging process should be doing strength training. Let's see why.

Sarcopenia

Sarcopenia is the loss of lean body mass, mainly muscle, with age. As people grow older, they lose muscle, and this process can start at a relatively young age, even by age 30, although it's rarely noticeable then. By age 50, however, this muscle loss becomes quite noticeable, and proceeds at a rate of up to 1% a year; the average muscle loss between the ages of 50 and 70 is about 30% of all muscle, and from the ages of 70 to 80, another 20 to 30% is lost, such that by age 80, the average person can lose fully 50% of all muscle that he or she had when younger.[53] Gone.

Plenty of older men and women have managed to maintain a low level of body fat, but the vast majority of these people have stick figures, since they've lost so much muscle. It's particularly noticeable in the buttocks, which in young people have a large muscle mass, but in older people all but disappears or is replaced by fat. A decent diet can help keep body fat at bay, but will do little in the way of retaining and building muscle.

This muscle loss is extremely bad for health, and contributes to many of the maladies of old age. Since muscle is such a metabolically active tissue, taking up glucose and amino acids, burning energy, and contributing to energy and nutrient levels, loss of muscle contributes to diabetes, obesity, and frailty. These conditions are extremely common in old age and contribute to many of the life difficulties of the elderly.

Sarcopenia is also an important public health problem, since almost everyone who gets old develops it to some degree, and it leads to weakness and inability to lead a normal daily life. Frail elderly people are much more prone to becoming disabled, to being unable to do normal tasks and movements without help, and to falling down with consequent breaking of bones and other damage. When this happens, elderly people often end up in nursing homes when they become unable to take care of themselves. Good muscle strength and mass is critical to living an independent life in old age; if you can't even get up from a chair or walk down the hall because of weakness, then life on your own is going to be tough.

Hip fractures are a major consequence of falls, and the falls themselves are largely a consequence of low muscle strength and inability to control movement – a minor tripping or getting a little off-balance, something young people with lots of muscle easily recover from, turns into a fall in the elderly. Hip fractures in turn are a major mortality risk, with women over 65 who had a hip fracture being twice as likely to die within a year as those without a fracture.[54]

For good health and quality of life in older age, avoidance of sarcopenia and retention of as much muscle as possible is essential.

One cause of muscle wasting in old age lies in the deterioration of mitochondria, which are small organelles within cells that are responsible for energy production. They are often referred to as the powerhouses of the cell. With aging, mitochondria become less efficient, are unable to generate energy as well, and emit large numbers of free radicals that damage the surrounding tissue. All of this can contribute to sarcopenia.

Physical activity can almost completely prevent this deterioration of the mitochondria.[55] In a group of people aged 21 to 95, no association of age with mitochondrial function was found, but there was a significant correlation with level of physical activity.

What this shows is that, at least in respect to mitochondrial function, disuse and lack of exercise may be much more important determinants of the pathology of aging than is age itself.

Use it or lose it, they use to say. (Maybe they still do.) Much of the physiological deterioration of aging comes from disuse and atrophy, not from the mere passing of years.

Illness accelerates muscle loss

In old age, illness occurs much more frequently, and this leads to long-term immobilization such as sitting, or spending large amounts of time in bed, or hospitalization. When someone is bedridden or hospitalized, muscle deteriorates and is lost at an alarming rate. If something isn't done to counteract it, the loss could be permanent.

In an experiment, healthy older people, average age 67, were placed on ten days of strict bed rest, and lost about 1 kg (2.2 pounds) of muscle mass from their lower extremities alone.[56] When the upper body is included in an analysis like this, muscle loss would be much greater, and even more so when elderly people in ill health are considered, and when they're in bed longer than ten days. The results could be catastrophic for health and quality of life.

Many patients in the hospital are undernourished, and this adds to the problem of muscle loss.[57] Sick people may have little appetite; add to this the fact that most hospital food is low-protein processed junk that's high in sugar, which sucks at retaining and building muscle, and you've got a 1-2 punch for muscle loss.

When people become critically ill due to trauma, burns, cancer, or infection, their metabolism makes higher demands for amino acids, which are the building blocks of proteins. The body will break down muscle to get them – which is known as a state of catabolism – and muscle loss, sometimes a massive amount, takes place. Given all this, it's not surprising that critically ill people who have a greater amount of muscle have a better survival rate than those with less muscle. So in these cases of critical illness, previous strength training can be a genuine lifesaver.[58] After the event, strength training can help recover the loss.

People live longer than ever now, making muscle loss more of a problem than ever. Unfortunately, hardly any older people are encouraged by their doctors or by anyone else to engage in strength training. They're just told that walking is enough, or given a set of very lame exercises like stretching or standing at the side of a chair and moving their legs. Official government guidelines even classify things like gardening as exercise. While these things are an improvement on being completely sedentary, they do not qualify as exercise in any meaningful sense of the word.

Just because your doctor or the U.S. government says something doesn't make it true.

Being totally sedentary is at one extreme of physical activity, and if you're sedentary enough, it could cause muscle loss at nearly as great a rate as does being bedridden. Walking is a step up, but strength training is arguably the total opposite of being sedentary and is the most efficient way to maintain and build muscle.

Osteoporosis

Osteoporosis – the more severe condition – and osteopenia are pathologies in which bone density becomes lower and bones become more liable to breaking. These conditions often accompany loss of muscle. Strength training increases bone mineral density.[59] Some other forms of exercise, such as walking or jogging, may increase bone density in the legs and hips, but do nothing for the rest of the body. A few forms of exercise, such as swimming or cycling, may do little or nothing for bones. Strength training helps bones in the whole body become denser and stronger.

In contrast, supplements such as calcium have a poor record in strengthening bone, because osteoporosis doesn't occur due to lack of calcium, but to the disuse of bones that comes with lack of physical activity in aging. Calcium supplements may actually increase the risk of death, because unless the body directs all ingested calcium to the bones, some of it heads for the lining of the arteries, leading to or exacerbating atherosclerosis, the narrowing and hardening of the arteries.

Osteoporosis is not caused by insufficient calcium. It's caused by disuse, a lack of load placed on the bones.

Bone has in common with muscle the fact that it continually breaks down and builds up; if the breaking down exceeds building up, net loss of bone occurs.

Astronauts who spend extended time in space suffer bone loss from doing so. This happens because of lack of gravity; astronauts are weightless in space, so no weight bears on their bones, which need regular stress to stay in good shape. This example shows the importance of weight-bearing exercise for good bone health. To avoid the bone fate of astronauts, regular weight-bearing exercise, most notably strength training, will ensure that bones remain strong and not brittle.

Wolff's law was developed by the 19th century German anatomist Julius Wolff, who noted that in a healthy human or animal, bone adapts to the load under which it is placed. If a bone endures a heavier than usual load, it remodels itself in order to withstand the load. (This is exactly what muscle does.) The reverse also occurs; if not enough load is placed on a bone, it becomes lighter and weaker, since any tissue is costly to maintain at the metabolic level. A mechanical signal, in this case a weighted load, is translated into biochemical signals that tell the bone cells to build more bone.

Weight placed on the bones is not the whole story for good bone health. Muscles are attached to bones, and when they contract, place a force on them. Some researchers believe that muscular contractions are the largest source of loads placed on bone.[60] There are strong correlations between grip strength and bone mass, both in healthy and ill people, and between body mass and bone strength also.

The maintenance of a healthy amount of muscle mass as well as muscle strength are crucial in staving off osteoporosis and keeping bones healthy.

A recent trial done in Australia, LIFTMOR (Lifting Intervention for Training Muscle and Osteoporosis Rehabilitation), enrolled a group of 28 post-menopausal women into a resistance training program; a paper about their study actually used the words "heavy resistance training". The program consisted of 8 months of twice weekly weightlifting sessions, 30 minutes each session. The sessions were supervised by a trainer. A control group performed a low-intensity workout routine at home, of the kind that are normally recommended for seniors.[61]

The resistance training group solidly increased bone mineral density, while the control group *lost* bone mass. Compliance, that is, the willingness to show up for exercise and continue the training, was greater than 87%, which is much better than the dismal < 50% normally found for prescribed exercise. Importantly, the study's authors state, "There were no injuries."

The women worked out with barbells and dumbbells, just like real weightlifters do, and they performed deadlifts, squats, shoulder presses, in short, the main compound exercises, again like real weightlifters. (These exercises are discussed in the chapter on basic strength training.) You can watch a video of their exercise sessions **here**.

The researchers concluded, "Brief supervised HiPRT [high-intensity progressive resistance training] with impact loading is a safe and effective exercise therapy for postmenopausal women with low to very low bone mass."

Funny, but you almost never hear about resistance training being recommended to fight osteoporosis. That's a shame, as osteoporosis is such a great scourge of old age, leading to disability and death.

Another problem often seen in aging is bad backs. Training reduces osteoporosis and can therefore restore thickness and strength to the vertebrae of the back as well. One often sees people, men and women both, who although lean enough, walk with bent spines. Sometimes this may be because people bend their backs to avoid pain. It can also be due to compression fracture, a collapse of one of the vertebrae in the spine, which causes the entire spine to become bent.

Strength training reinforces good posture by strengthening the muscles and tendons that support the spine. It also does this because good form is required in strength training, and that includes good posture. And by strengthening the bone in the spine, compression fractures become less likely.

If you strength train into old age, it can help you keep your spine healthy and allow you to maintain a healthy, straight back, so important not just for health but for appearance and attractiveness.

The causes of sarcopenia

As we age, the physiological processes of our bodies become deregulated, and we can no longer maintain normal homeostasis, that is, the maintenance of normal function. One of the most important of these processes is an increase in inflammation. This is such a prominent characteristic of aging that a term has been coined for it: "inflammaging".[62]

Low-level inflammation of the kind seen in aging is an important cause of sarcopenia.

In a normal, healthy person, muscle tissue breaks down and builds up cyclically and daily, depending on factors like the last time we ate, how much protein we ate, whether we're getting enough calories, and physical activity. Lack of food and being sedentary cause a net breakdown in muscle, whereas being fed and performing exercise cause a net increase in muscle synthesis.

In young people, this cycle proceeds normally, but in older people, the cycle flattens out.

The consequence of increased inflammation in the elderly is *anabolic resistance*, which occurs when a stimulus, such as exercise or protein, does not cause as great an increase in muscle synthesis (anabolism) as it would in a younger person.

While an older person may have the same degree of daily muscle breakdown as in a younger person, they fail to build the muscle back up again to the same level.

When anabolic resistance goes on long enough, and the person fails to build muscle at the proper rate, a net loss of muscle follows, and if this goes on long enough, frank sarcopenia occurs.

The good news is that resistance training can remedy anabolic resistance.[63]

Elderly people who lift weights show a robust response to it, and gain strength and muscle readily.

Anabolic resistance appears to be related to insulin sensitivity as well. A recent study took a number of older (average age 71, which is not really elderly by my lights) men and women and put them on a resistance training program for a mere eight weeks. Their glucose tolerance, a measure of insulin sensitivity, markedly improved, as did their strength and muscle aerobic capacity.[64]

Older people often, in fact usually, have impaired insulin sensitivity, or increased insulin resistance, and overweight and obesity is very often seen in conjunction with it. One study took a group of sedentary, overweight men and women, aged 60 to 80 years, and divided them into two groups, one for weight loss, the other for weight loss and resistance training.[65] The results strongly favored the resistance training group.

Hemoglobin A1C (HbA1C), a measure of blood sugar control, fell much more in the resistance training group, nearly ten times more. Both groups lost a similar amount of fat, but the training group gained lean body mass, while the group that did no strength training lost lean mass, which is unhealthy and even dangerous for older people. So, an intensive weight training program, with its beneficial effects on blood sugar control, muscular strength, and lean body mass, is a very useful component of treatment for older diabetics.

A review of strength training for elderly people[66] notes that it

- is an effective intervention for sarcopenia by increasing muscle mass and strength
- can increase endurance performance
- can decrease blood pressure
- reduces insulin resistance
- reduces total and abdominal fat
- increases resting metabolic rate
- prevents loss of bone mineral density

- reduces risk factors for falls
- may reduce pain and improve function in osteoarthritis

Strength training: is there anything it can't do?

A dramatic example of the power of weightlifting can be seen in an intervention protocol done on patients with hip fractures.[67] You thought that only young, buff guys lifted weights? Hip fracture patients are typically old, frail women with osteoporosis and low muscle mass. Their lack of muscle and frailty leads to a decreased ability to stand, walk, and stay balanced. Then at some point they lose their balance or trip, fall down to the ground, and break a hip. Wrists are another frequently broken bone during falls.

The group on which the resistance training intervention was done consisted of 124 patients admitted over a several year period to a hospital for surgical repair of a hip fracture. They were compared to another group of patients receiving "usual care", just standard medical and surgical treatment. The main intervention was "high-intensity progressive resistance training", supervised by a trainer, two days a week for 12 months. "Progressive" in this context refers to increasing the amount of weight and/or training level of the participants as they get stronger, so that they don't reach a plateau and continue to improve. The patients also received nutritional and psychological support and treatment for polypharmacy (excessive number of medications).

The results were astounding. Allow me to put them in boldface.

Risk of death was reduced by 81%.

Nursing home admissions were reduced by 84%.

Both groups, the intervention and the control group, received the same hospital care. Afterward, only the intervention group lifted weights, and that made all the difference to their lives.

It's an absolute shame that this type of intervention isn't standard care for patients like these. Instead, we just send them home and allow large numbers of them to die.

Falls are a huge source of injury, disability and death. According to the Centers for Disease Control, in the United States some 2.5 million people are treated in emergency rooms for falls every year.[68] One out of every five falls causes a serious injury such as broken bones and head injuries. (This means that the number of falls greatly exceeds 2.5 million a year, since only the serious ones are deemed worthy of medical attention.) Over 700,000 people a year are hospitalized because of falls, mostly due to head injuries or hip fractures, and over 95% of hip fractures are caused by falls. Falls cost over $34 billion annually, mainly from hospitalization.

Among the causes of falls, the most important are lower body weakness, and difficulty with walking and maintaining balance. While neurological deterioration can be involved, *lack of muscular strength leading to poor balance and difficulty in walking is the main cause of falls*.

Hence it can be seen that declining muscular strength is a huge cause of injury, disability, and death in the elderly. To the extent that the elderly are prescribed any exercise at all, the prescribed exercises are normally very ineffective ones that entail standing next to a chair and extending a leg or arm or similar exercises. These will do little to improve muscular strength. They amount to little more than a holding action against long-term decline.

While the frail elderly may need to start slowly and of course be medically supervised, a strength training program remains the best way to abolish frailty and lower the odds of falls occurring.

Elderly, infirm people, as well as their loved ones, should not overlook the power of strength training. An older, frail person cannot of course just go sign up at the gym or get a bench with weights at home, but needs a supervised program of exercise, whether with machines (Nautilus or similar) or free weights (barbells and dumbbells).

Medicare currently pays for extensive rehabilitation programs, so if you or your family members have had, e.g., a broken or replaced hip, or heart attack or stroke, that may be an option. In order to qualify for Medicare, skilled nursing facilities must offer physical therapy at least 5 days a week. Even if extensive rehabilitation including strength training is available, that doesn't at all mean that a doctor will be aware of it and prescribe it. So taking the initiative in getting an elderly person into a program like this may be required. Don't wait for the medical system to initiate, because it often will not.

In my experience, the type of therapy offered in rehabilitation centers can be incredibly minimal. After a major medical event, minimal may of course be all that someone is capable of. But the facility should have the ability to escalate the therapy into progressive (increasing) resistance training, and that option may be hard to find. If you're looking for a skilled nursing or long-term care facility, it may be best to shop around to find one that offers resistance training, along with skilled therapists or trainers that can assist.

An inpatient rehabilitation facility (IRF) usually has more intensive and varied therapy for patients than a skilled nursing facility (SNF), and Medicare may pay for this. Patients who reside in IRFs have better outcomes than those in SNFs; for instance, 81% of IRF residents returned home, compared to only 45% of SNF patients; 76% of IRF patients were walking independently on discharge, compared to only 31% of SNF patients.[69] Intensive rehabilitation, then, has about double the chance of an excellent outcome for the ill elderly person than does skilled nursing.

Resistance training strengthens the brain

Dementia and cognitive decline are two problems of aging that everyone would like to avoid at all costs. Fortunately, exercise and particularly resistance training can improve cognition and fight dementia.

Exercise in general has robust effects on cognition, that is, the ability to think properly. It can even increase brain volume, and it seems to do much of this through an increase in brain-derived neurotrophic factor, or BDNF, a molecule important to both brain and muscle function. Resistance training induces a robust increase in BDNF.[70]

With one session of strength training, BDNF levels rise, then fall back to normal. But with repeated training sessions, the increase in BDNF becomes greater than at first, and when it declines after a session, the basal level is now higher than before. This indicates that a regular strength training program augments the BDNF response. The fitter one becomes in terms of muscular strength, the greater the rise in both acute and chronic levels of BDNF.

In older people with mild cognitive impairment, which is considered to be a forerunner of dementia, resistance training twice a week for six months improved "selective attention/conflict resolution, associative memory, and regional patterns of functional brain plasticity, compared to aerobic exercise, which improved only physical function.[71] In Alzheimer's, associative memory decline is a hallmark of the disease, so resistance training has the ability to help prevent this disease. It looks as if resistance training better prevents dementia and Alzheimer's than aerobic exercise does.

There is robust evidence that increased physical activity can improve memory and even increase brain volume in older people. Strength training has the extra benefit of increasing strength, lean mass, and metabolic health., besides the cognitive benefits.

As with cancer, many people mistakenly believe that dementia and memory loss just strike at random and that there's little one can do about it. Nothing could be further from the truth. The brain is a biological mechanism, an organ that obeys the same rules that other organs in the body obey. When you get your body in better shape, as through strength training, all of your organs become healthier, including the brain.

Exercise of any kind can help prevent dementia. Older people who engaged in four or more different kinds of physical activity have a risk of dementia only about half that of people who engage in one or fewer kinds of activity.[72] Keep in mind that, in research jargon, "physical activity" doesn't necessarily refer to exercise as such, only activities that result in moving around, such as gardening or housework. Actual exercise is even more powerful at preventing cognitive decline and dementia.

The brain, like skeletal muscle, is plastic, that is, it can change size and structure depending on environmental influences on it such as exercise. Experiments in animals have demonstrated that exercise changes gene expression in the brain, which leads to changed function. Changed for the better.[73]

Strength training slows aging

As we've seen above, strength training (resistance training, weightlifting) powerfully prevents several of the most prominent symptoms of aging: sarcopenia or muscle wasting, osteoporosis, and dementia.

Aging also makes a person prone to lots of other illnesses and debilities as well. Obesity, diabetes, heart disease, cancer: older people have increased rates of all of these diseases. As we've covered in other chapters, strength training can substantially cut the risk of some of these, and for others nearly eliminate them altogether.

Obviously, if you're not quite old yet and don't have any of these maladies, strength training can keep you from ever getting them.

Takeaway points

- Exercise fights aging, but aerobic exercise doesn't prevent and may exacerbate muscle loss

- Virtually everyone suffers muscle loss (sarcopenia), and this starts at relatively young ages
- Muscle loss leads to dependence, frailty, and nursing homes
- Illness and bed rest increase muscle loss
- Lack of weight-bearing exercise can lead to osteoporosis
- Strength training prevents muscle loss and osteoporosis
- Strength training can lower death rates of hip-fracture patients and keep them out of nursing homes
- Strength training increases BDNF and can prevent dementia

Chapter 6: Strength training increases testosterone in men

Testosterone is a steroid hormone that makes men what they are: it gives them the secondary sex characteristics of a deep voice, abundant body hair, and larger, stronger muscles, and it affects behavior too. Women also have testosterone, but men have about ten times as much.

Testosterone – the standard shorthand for testosterone is "T", which I'll be using a lot from now on – is also responsible for the sex drive, and increasing or decreasing levels of T increase or decrease the sex drive. As men age, T levels almost invariably decline, leading to symptoms such as low sex drive, muscular weakness and fatigue, and depression. Some "exceptionally healthy" men appear not to experience any decline in T, which questions whether a decline in T really is due to age, or whether other factors are more important, such as overall health, obesity, smoking, alcohol use, etc.[74]

T levels also have a strong reciprocal relation to obesity. Low T can lead to obesity, and vice versa. Testosterone replacement therapy (TRT), which is the supplementation of T either through injections or gels, can have salutary effects on body composition, leading to less fat and more muscle.

Parallel to, or similar to, the decline in T seen in aging men is a long-term declining trend in T levels in *all* men. That is, an average young man of, say, 20, will today have lower T levels than a 20-year-old man of even a few decades ago, and the numbers are not small. Whereas a man a generation ago may have had a T level of 500, now it may be more like 400, a 20% drop. This phenomenon is seen in both the U.S. and in Europe.[75,76]

A number of factors have been implicated in this decline, such as obesity and environmental pollutants, especially so-called endocrine disruptors, which are estrogen-like compounds that stick around in the environment a long time. Endocrine disruptors can unfortunately be found in many common consumer personal care products, such as soaps, shampoos, and deodorants, as well as in packaging and plastics, so the risk of exposure is not remote. They can persist in the body for a long time after exposure, and accumulate with repeated exposure.

Lower levels of T can have serious health effects, including increased cardiovascular disease and worse mental health, including depression. A man with low T doesn't feel or in many cases look as masculine as a man with normal levels, and neither does he perform as well sexually or have as high a sex drive.

What if there were a simple solution to low T, would you be interested? What if a straightforward intervention that costs little (or even nothing) could raise your T levels, and at the same time improve your overall health, make you look better and give you miles more confidence, how would you feel about that?

As you may have guessed, the answer is resistance training, which has a robust effect in raising T levels, as well as increasing muscle mass, cardiovascular fitness, and decreasing depression.

One reason to choose resistance training over testosterone replacement therapy as a means to raise T is that many – probably most – doctors are very wary about prescribing TRT for their patients. The DEA has classified testosterone as a Schedule 3 Controlled Substance, meaning that it's considered to have a potential for abuse; any physician who prescribes it is subject to extra governmental scrutiny, especially if he prescribes it often.

Therefore, unless you have a very low T level, say under 300, your doctor is unlikely to prescribe it for you. Men can have symptoms of low T at levels much higher than this, so what do you do when you're feeling depressed, are overweight, maybe have some erectile dysfunction, but your T levels are deemed too high for supplementation, and your doctor refuses to prescribe it?

You start a weightlifting program, that's what you do.

In a study designed to understand the hormonal response to weightlifting, two groups of men, 30 and 62 years old respectively, participated in a 10-week program of heavy resistance training.[77] Both groups responded robustly with an increase in T. Both basal levels and immediate post-training levels increased. Growth hormone levels also increased, as would be expected in cases where resistance training increased muscle mass, which it did in this study. IGF-1 levels were unchanged.

Cortisol, an anti-inflammatory hormone with catabolic properties – that is, it breaks down tissue, including muscle – was strongly lowered with ten weeks of training. This indicates that the training lowered inflammation, and the body did not require as much cortisol as before; this is a strong anti-aging effect.

As we've noted in previous chapters, resistance training is the best exercise for combating obesity, since muscular strength and muscle mass have a strong inverse association with obesity and with the illnesses that accompany it. And obesity is strongly associated with low T. Therefore, to treat both obesity and low T, lift weights.

Low T seen in obesity is associated with insulin resistance and development of the metabolic syndrome, which is the prelude to type 2 diabetes.[78] In turn, this increases the incidence of cardiovascular disease and erectile dysfunction.

In short, if you are man and are obese, you can expect illness to come calling, partly due to T levels that are lower than in lean men. Poor morning erections, low sexual desire, and erectile dysfunction are all associated with low T.

Testosterone comes in two flavors, protein-bound, and unbound. Both taken together are referred to as total T, and unbound is known as free T. Low levels of free T are strongly associated with muscle wasting—

sarcopenia.[79] Men with low free T are nearly twice as likely to have sarcopenia as men with normal levels.

As for anti-aging effects of testosterone, consider the recently reported experiments in so-called parabiosis, in which scientists graft the circulatory systems of two mice together. When a young mouse is paired with an old mouse, the old one shows strong rejuvenating effects, including increased muscle mass. It turns out that T is required for these effects: no T, no increase in muscle.[80]

Mostly, the effects of resistance training on T levels seem to be attributable to a change in body composition: less fat and more muscle.

Contrast the effects of endurance training — running and other aerobic exercise – on testosterone levels. Men who chronically perform high levels of endurance training can have decreased T levels, so much so that it's been termed "the exercise-hypogonadal male condition".[81] Endurance training has "significant detrimental effects upon reproductive hormonal profiles in men." Endurance exercise may also cause lower sperm counts. This condition seems to be mainly confined to men who have done chronic endurance training for many years.

If you're a man and out there cranking out a lot of weekly running mileage, then you could be setting yourself up for a bout of ill health through low T levels, not the good health you'd hoped for.

The difference in T levels between strength trainers and runners could have much to do with their respective body types: muscular vs skinny.

A comparison of T levels in triathletes, cyclists, and swimmers found that only the triathletes and cyclists had lower levels, leading the authors to suggest that the endurance component of exercise may be the causative factor.[82]

Weightlifting, confidence, and self-esteem

Almost any type of exercise can help fight depression. People who exercise regularly have lower rates of depression and anxiety. If I had one piece of advice to give to anyone feeling blue, it would be to exercise, and especially, train with weights.

Little actual research has been done on the effect of resistance training and how it affects personality, but going by my own experience as well as that of many others I've talked to, becoming proficient at lifting weights and developing a better body type profoundly increases self-esteem and confidence. No doubt that is partly due to direct effects effects on the brain, such as increasing blood flow, levels of neurotransmitters, and brain-derived neurotrophic factor.

The emotions function as a sensor that interprets to us how we should react to certain events, including events inside the body. Think of your state of mind when you're ill: you feel down, don't want to do anything much. This emotion is your mind interpreting that your body needs rest, and this state is known as sickness behavior, which is also associated with depression. Depressed people may feel fatigued, unmotivated, and have many physical symptoms of illness.

Ill health is strongly associated with depressed mood; for instance, people with heart disease are much more likely to be depressed than those without. So keeping oneself healthy is a good first step in avoiding depression and anxiety.

For men especially, weightlifting has a tremendous positive effect on confidence and feelings of well-being. Many of my friends are, like myself, almost addicted to lifting. Much of this can be attributed to the instantaneous mood lift that a bout of hard weightlifting gives.

Building muscle powerfully boosts self-confidence. People begin to look at you in a new light, they see you as more worthy of respect. More muscular men are of course seen as more masculine, and this means that a man who lifts becomes more attractive to women. In fact, if a man came to me for advice on how to make himself more attractive to women, the first thing I'd tell him is to get into the gym and start lifting. Everything else can wait.

The musician Henry Rollins (Black Flag) has written powerfully of how lifting weights boosted his self-confidence and self-esteem.[83] When he was in high school, he felt out of place, he was threatened and bullied, and teachers told him that he would never amount to anything. He writes, "I hated myself all the time." Then a teacher who was a military veteran took a liking to him and basically commanded Rollins to start lifting weights. It transformed him. He went from a skinny, bullied adolescent to a strong, self-confident man.

"It wasn't until my late twenties that I learned that by working out I had given myself a great gift. I learned that nothing good comes without work and a certain amount of pain. When I finish a set that leaves me shaking, I know more about myself. When something gets bad, I know it can't be as bad as that workout.

"I used to fight the pain, but recently this became clear to me: pain is not my enemy; it is my call to greatness. But when dealing with the Iron, one must be careful to interpret the pain correctly. Most injuries involving the Iron come from ego. I once spent a few weeks lifting weight that my body wasn't ready for and spent a few months not picking up anything heavier than a fork. Try to lift what you're not prepared to and the Iron will teach you a little lesson in restraint and self-control.

"I have never met a truly strong person who didn't have self-respect."

The overweight and obese can have low self-esteem and self-confidence. It seems that many obese people feel ashamed of the way they look, and you can imagine how such a feeling of inner shame affects one's interactions with other people and the world. I myself was somewhat overweight, when I was a teenager, and when I lost the weight through a combination of weightlifting and dieting, my self-confidence went way up, and my interactions with girls became much more successful. Losing fat and gaining muscle through strength training provide a potent boost to one's mental outlook.

Do women really like muscular bodies in their men? Obfuscating this question is the fact that the reaction of many women to the prototypical Mr. Universe contestant is "no thanks". But those guys are at the extreme end of a spectrum of male body types, and anyway, it's unlikely that many men will come to look like that without years of daily hard work in the gym along with some performance enhancing drugs. But as for the enhanced muscularity and lower body fat that men will get when they lift weights, yes, women do like that.[84] It's science.

Boys and girls, women, and weightlifting

Many boys, especially teenagers, become interested in lifting weights and adding muscle as part of their rite of passage into manhood. Hopefully, many of them will retain their gym habits for life. But unfortunately, there's a movement afoot to discourage boys and young men from strength training. Yes, I find it hard to believe too, but apparently some people believe that weightlifting encourages something called "toxic masculinity" in boys and men.

In contrast, I believe that lifting weights will do nothing but good for boys and young men. They will improve their bodies and health, develop more self-confidence, and gain camaraderie with other boys and men in their situation.

Many associations of exercise professionals have issued position papers on resistance training for children and adolescents.[85] The general consensus is that, provided the training is tailored for the different needs of this population, and that it is properly designed and supervised, children and adolescents can benefit from resistance training.

What about weightlifting and women? I've covered the benefits of weightlifting for women in another chapter, but here let's just say that strength training can have the same good effects on women in terms of mood and self-confidence that they have for men.

Gaining muscle is difficult for women, but the fat loss that comes from strength training will benefit them greatly.

Men find slender women attractive. Does that need to be proved by science? Probably not, but it has been.[86] Men all over the world, even blind men who presumably have never been acculturated with images of slender women, prefer women within a certain narrow waist-hip ratio.

As we've seen, weightlifting should always accompany all weight loss efforts, or you risk losing muscle, which is deleterious for health. Weightlifting simply has the best record of any exercise for fat loss and for keeping waist circumference low, and this is one of the best ways to improve one's appearance and get the self-confidence that goes with it.

Takeaway points

- Testosterone gives men their secondary sex characteristics as well as sex drive and function
- Testosterone declines with age, unless you're "exceptionally healthy"
- There's a long-term decline in testosterone levels among men
- Resistance training can increase T levels
- Weightlifting instills confidence and self-esteem, and makes men and women more attractive

Chapter 7: Drawbacks of aerobic exercise

Aerobic exercise is an inefficient way to go about getting into shape. As we've seen in other chapters, it doesn't do much for fat loss, and if combined with any kind of low-calorie diet, can lead to losing muscle along with the fat, a situation that should be avoided at all costs. Muscle loss decreases the metabolic rate and makes it more difficult to lose fat and sustain the loss without regain.

Aerobic exercise is also inefficient at improving cardiorespiratory fitness, because it typically operates at a relatively low, steady-state level of oxygen and energy demand. Higher intensity exercise is much more efficient at improving fitness, and both strength training and high-intensity training fall into this category. As one wag put it, the best idea of "cardio" is lifting weights faster.

In addition to inefficiencies in fat loss and conditioning, aerobic exercise has some major pitfalls, even dangers. It can harm you in ways that strength training will not, the reason for this mostly being related to the longer times that people perform aerobic exercise, leading to a syndrome of overuse. Some of the dangers of aerobics can be relatively minor, such as shin splints; others can be major, such as scarring of the heart or death from a heart attack.

Joints

One of the most common problems seen in aerobic exercise is injury to a joint, and the most common joint affected is the knee. Running, especially, causes great, repeated force to be placed on the knee joint, and if done enough can lead to damage. This could apply to any kind of running, such as on treadmills in the gym. If someone is overweight or obese, then the force put on the knee is even greater, since body weight is the main determinant of that force.

A review of studies that looked at the putative connection between running and joint injuries found a wide range of the incidence of lower extremity injuries associated with running, ranging from about 20% to 80% of runners.[87] In some studies in which non-lower-extremity injuries were also included, the incidence of injury from running increased all the way up to 92%. Personally I don't like the odds of a sport or form of exercise that will give me that high a chance of injury, potentially even a crippling one. I don't know whether that risk rate includes being bitten by a dog, but that's actually a real problem for runners. I've come very close to it.

The most common site of injury that these studies found was the knee, with incidence ranging from 7 to 50%. Other common sites of injuries were shins, feet and toes, the muscles of the upper leg including thigh and hamstrings. Somewhat less common were injuries to the ankle, hips, and groin.

Risk factors for injuring oneself while running included greater age – no surprise there. Female runners were more likely than male to injure their hips. Taller men were more likely than shorter men to be injured.

What mainly causes these injuries is overuse, and this is inherent to aerobic exercise, since it substitutes time for intensity. Instead of several sprints lasting for between 10 and 30 seconds each, even casual runners may pound the pavement for 30 minutes at a time several times a week. More serious runners may run quite a bit more than that, increasing the chances of injury.

These types of overuse injuries can sometimes be serious, causing great pain and needing surgery to correct.

What about running on a treadmill, is that safer? In 2014, around 24,400 treadmill-associated injuries were reported in emergency departments in the U.S., compared to a total of 62,700 injuries reported for all exercise equipment, including weights, golf clubs, and trampolines.[88] Note that the numbers are for ER visits only, so many of these incidents could be due to things like falling off a treadmill rather than overuse injuries. In fairness, it's difficult to make sense of these numbers without knowing how many people were on treadmills, or out playing golf, etc. Stationary cycles and elliptical machines are safer than treadmills because they are entirely human-powered, whereas the motor that runs a treadmill can throw you off the machine.

In the U.S. in 2013, 4,735 pedestrians and 743 bicyclists were killed by cars and trucks.[89] How many of those were out for the exercise, no one knows, just as the relative safety of cycling and walking isn't known (since we'd have to know number of miles ridden or walked among other things). But the number of people hit by cars while lifting weights was presumably very low, so there's that.

The effects of aerobics on the heart are not all good

Besides mechanical injuries as discussed above, aerobic exercise can have bad systemic effects on health, especially when done to excess.

Now, we know that people who exercise have better health than sedentary people. That is not in dispute, and it's certainly not my aim here to discourage exercise. I'm interested in a couple of things: one, to show that strength and high-intensity training have more advantages and fewer drawbacks than steady-state aerobic exercise; and two, to show that aerobic exercise may not be the 100% safe cure-all with no important side effects that most people have been encouraged to believe.

Jogging is a common form of aerobics, perhaps the most performed after walking. Joggers have around a 70% lower mortality rate than sedentary people.[90]

But (from the same study, the Copenhagen City Heart Study) light joggers had the lowest mortality rate, followed by moderate and strenuous. That's right, more jogging resulted in a higher death rate, a result contrary to received opinion. This means that there's "a U-shaped association between all-cause mortality and dose of jogging as calibrated by pace, quantity, and frequency of jogging. Light and moderate joggers have lower mortality than sedentary non-joggers, whereas *strenuous joggers have a mortality rate not statistically different from that of the sedentary group.*"[My emphasis.]

Just from the Copenhagen data, it appears that the dose of aerobic exercise that maximizes health is relatively low, amounting to relatively slow jogging two or three times a week.

Fitness does not equal health. It's entirely possible to overdo exercise, and to become less healthy by doing more of it. Just because someone has the VO_2max of an elite Olympic athlete does not mean that that person has therefore maximized his health. This truth is all but ignored or unknown these days, with many people mistakenly believing that they must perform a strenuous workout such as distance running daily in order to be as healthy as possible. No, many "extreme exercisers" should *reduce* the amount of exercise they do in order to become healthier.

How much exercise conduces to ill health is an open question at this point, but it doesn't seem to be all that high, at least when it comes to jogging and perhaps other forms of aerobic activity.

Extreme aerobic exercise such as distance running could lead to heart disease, chronic fatigue, and perhaps even cancer.

A group of 102 marathon runners were examined for "late gadolinium enhancement", or LGE, a radiological term that shows the extent of damage to the myocardium of the heart, and which is associated with both coronary artery disease and with sudden cardiac death.[91] A group of age-matched controls, non-runners, were also examined.

The marathon runners had *three times the incidence of LGE* compared to controls—12% of the marathoners vs 4% of controls. These runners had no symptoms of heart disease. The extent of LGE was related to the number of marathons that each runner had completed, which suggests that it was extreme exercise that caused the heart damage.

The marathon runners also had a higher level of coronary artery calcification, an important measure of risk for cardiovascular disease, than controls that were matched by Framingham risk factors – for things like cholesterol, blood pressure, and so on. Again, this suggests that exercise was a causative factor for coronary artery calcification.

So, extreme exercise can result in worse health, including heart disease, than no exercise at all. Yet these marathoners undoubtedly had very high fitness levels – a VO$_2$max through the roof – combined with hidden heart disease.

Lifelong veteran endurance athletes don't appear to have great heart health either. In 12 of these athletes who were examined, and compared against both age-matched controls and younger veteran endurance athletes who had no signs of illness, a full 50% of the veteran athletes showed signs of myocardial fibrosis, compared to none of the controls or younger athletes.[92] The development of myocardial fibrosis can lead to heart arrhythmias which, depending on the particular type, can be fatal.

A quote from this study speaks volumes:

"The prevalence of LGE [myocardial fibrosis] in veteran athletes was not associated with age, height, weight, or body surface area, but was significantly associated with the number of years spent training, number of competitive marathons, and ultraendurance (>50 miles) marathons completed. An unexpectedly high prevalence of myocardial fibrosis (50%) was observed in healthy, asymptomatic, lifelong veteran male athletes, compared with zero cases in age-matched veteran controls and young athletes. These data suggest a link between lifelong endurance exercise and myocardial fibrosis that requires further investigation."

There was a direct association of the amount, duration, and number of years of running with myocardial fibrosis.

If you're a runner, be advised that more is not necessarily better. We don't know at what level the benefits of aerobic exercise turn into detriments, but it doesn't appear to be terribly high.

Extreme exercise has been reported to be a risk factor for chronic fatigue, although the numbers are not known, and adequate rest and nutrition may resolve this problem.

That extreme aerobic exercise can result in joint, heart, and immune damage appears to be due to the relatively long duration of such exercise. Getting the heart rate to a very high level for long periods of time may stress it in a way that nature did not intend. In contrast, in strength or high-intensity training, the heart rate becomes elevated but for much shorter periods of time.

Why should extreme aerobic exercise have this effect on health? It comes down to what type of environment humans are adapted to. In the long course of human evolution, did humans regularly run for an hour or more without stopping and with an elevated heart rate? Probably not. Humans are apex predators, and it's normally prey animals that have the ability to run long distances. Predators run fast and for a short time: sprints. Most hunter-gatherer physical activity appears to be walking, sprinting, throwing (spears and rocks), climbing, and so on. To my knowledge, no group of hunter-gatherers has been shown to be distance runners, though they certainly walk long distances.

Then again, are humans adapted to strength training? Hunter-gatherers don't do bench presses either. But weightlifting and other forms of strength training cause an increase in muscle growth, and the fact that humans can respond physiologically in this way argues for a much better alignment of this kind of training with our evolutionary past.

Strength training also seems to be harder to overdo. With extreme aerobic exercise, the heart rate may be elevated for periods of time that damage it, but the runner experiences no signals (pain, for instance) that tell him to stop. If the runner's legs are still going strong, that's all he or she knows. Strength training doesn't have that problem, because the exercises, while intense, or rather because of their intensity, last but a short duration until the exerciser is forced to stop due to muscle fatigue or being out of breath.

To be sure, some weightlifters overdo it and may have problems such as inflamed and painful tendons, or in extreme cases using very heavy weights, they can damage their joints and backs. The frequency and difference in rate between the health problems in extreme aerobic exercisers vs extreme weightlifters is not known with precision, but some studies have shown an injury rate in bodybuilders of between 0.24 to 5.5 injuries per 1000 hours of training, while in runners the figure is 2.5 to 12.1 injuries per 1000 hours.[93]

In any case, the use of anabolic steroids, the testosterone-like drugs that increase muscle growth, appear to be behind most of the serious health problems seen in the weightlifting world. These drugs can have serious side effects, especially when done to excess, and bodybuilders have died from their use, although what fraction of users has died is not known, and could be small for all anyone knows. Steroids have a large effect on recovery time, shortening it, and this allows the steroid user to exercise more often, hence boosting his ability to add muscle.

Takeaway points

- Aerobic exercise can damage joints
- The amount of aerobic exercise that promotes health and doesn't damage it appears to be lower than commonly thought
- When taken to an extreme, aerobic exercise can damage the heart
- Human beings may not be highly adapted to long-duration aerobic exercise
- Humans may be better adapted to strength and high-intensity training

Chapter 8: High-intensity training (HIT)

Previously in this book, we've discussed both the benefits of resistance training and how it is a much more effective and efficient way to train than traditional aerobics, or cardio. The idea behind cardio is that you exercise at a relatively low steady-state level for a relatively longer time. Jogging, for instance, has you move at a pace that you can hold for 20 or 30 minutes or even longer.

Low intensity, long duration exercise like jogging or other steady-state aerobic exercise is just a very inefficient way to improve cardiovascular fitness. Aerobics has the further drawback that you do not exercise the muscles in your entire body, and hence it does next to nothing to fight sarcopenia (muscle-wasting). It also has a poor record compared to resistance training when it comes to fat loss and waist size.

An exercise modality that appears to have many of the same beneficial effects as lifting weights is known as high-intensity training (HIT), or sometimes as high-intensity interval training (HIIT). (I prefer HIT, since it's much catchier, so that's what I'll use here.)

HIT as such has only come along relatively recently, although some athletes such as in track and field ("wind sprints") and in boxing (jump rope) have been doing forms of HIT for a long time. We don't have loads of academic studies on large numbers of people to gauge its effectiveness, but the studies that have been done show that those who do it get into good shape – and fast.

HIT can also work the entire musculature, and this means that it *will* fight muscle loss, unlike aerobics, and it therefore can be very helpful with fat loss. It may not be able to build muscle on quite the level as weightlifting does, but it does exercise all of them – depending on how you do it, which we'll discuss below – and strongly increases levels of mitochondria and other markers of excellent cardiovascular and metabolic fitness.

HIT has had excellent results in improving insulin sensitivity too.

What is HIT?

High-intensity training comes in almost as many forms as there are practitioners of it, but its essence lies in exercising at a very high intensity for short periods of time, punctuated by short rest intervals. (Those who know CrossFit will see many similarities to HIT: high intensity and a complete, whole-body workout. I'm not terribly fond of CrossFit because it appears to have a propensity to cause injuries, but that's another discussion.)

An example or two will serve to show what this is. Sprinting as fast as you can is a high-intensity exercise. For a sprint version of HIT, you could sprint all-out for 20 seconds, then walk until you get your breath back, which for beginners could be up to two minutes or more, then sprint again, walk again, and do this five times.

When you first do this, you will discover the real meaning of "all-out", and you'll be breathless after each sprint, and may even need a few days recovery time before you can do it again.

Consider another way to do HIT: with a jump rope. Jump fast for a minute (or less, if you can't go that long), then walk for a short break, and then do it again. Eight times should be plenty.

Calisthenics make for an excellent HIT workout, since using several types of body movement gets you closer to the whole-body workout you should be aiming for. For example, do push-ups as fast as you can for 30 seconds, rest for a short while, then do air squats (which we used to call deep knee bends) for 30 seconds, then rest, then burpees for 30 seconds, rest, then jump rope. Add jumping jacks, sprints, pull-ups or chin-ups, or whatever you feel like, so long as you get variety in the muscle groups you work. Do a total of ten sets, more as you get in better shape, and you've got one hell of a workout that takes only minutes, and that will improve your cardiovascular fitness immeasurably.

The exercise physiologists who developed HIT first used an exercise cycle in something called the Wingate test. In the Wingate test, a cycle is set to a certain resistance weight, and the cyclist cycles all-out for some period of time, usually 30 seconds. He then cycles at a leisurely pace for a few minutes, usually four, and then does another all-out 30 second bout, rest again, etc.

The physiologists discovered that this method of exercise could increase cardiorespiratory fitness incredibly quickly. For instance, in only two weeks, in six sessions of exercise, totaling only 12 to 18 minutes of all-out cycling – that's over the entire two-week period – skeletal muscle endurance capacity greatly increased.[94]

In a comparison with aerobic exercise similar to that recommended by public health experts, people performing HIT attained the same degree of aerobic fitness as more traditional exercise with *90% lower training volume and 67% less time*.

There goes the excuse that so many people use for not exercising: lack of time. If you have 10 minutes two or three times a week, you can get in shape using HIT.

However, there was one problem with the Wingate version of HIT: it's a difficult, intense, and very demanding exercise, and the researchers could only get young, healthy volunteers to do it. Others couldn't handle it, so exhausting it was.

So they set out to develop other ways to perform HIT, and to find out if they were as effective as the all-out assault of a Wingate test. And they were.

One way they did this was to decrease the absolute intensity of the exercise bouts, but increased them somewhat in duration, and shortened the rest intervals. One model was to cycle at 90% of maximum (instead of all-out), but for 60 seconds, interspersed with one-minute rest intervals, for a total of 10 times. This is still quite demanding, but much more palatable to most people.

One of the first researchers to investigate the possibilities of HIT was a man named Tabata in Japan.[95] Tabata and his colleagues compared traditional endurance training with a HIT workout, the form of which has come to be known as the Tabata workout. In this case, the Tabata workout was 7 to 8 bouts, 20 seconds each, of all-out cycling, with rest intervals of 10 seconds. This turned out to be even more effective than a huge amount of endurance exercise.

In effect, HIT substitutes intensity for time. The greater the intensity of the exercise, the lower the time needed to cause improvements in cardiorespiratory fitness.

The details of HIT as I've described are less important than the mere fact that you exercise at high intensity for from 20 to 60 seconds, rest, and do some more. Don't get bogged down too much in the details. Designing your own HIT routine is easy, or you can choose from an endless number of these routines that you can find online.

I'll discuss a few more practical HIT workouts below.

HIT, fat loss, and insulin sensitivity

HIT is, as I mentioned, too new to have a large body of research to back up extensive health claims for it, but so far, HIT looks highly promising.

HIT has been shown to be very effective in fat loss, reducing both subcutaneous and abdominal fat.[96] Continuous, steady-state aerobic exercise, such as jogging or treadmills, has very little to no capability in this regard. (As I've been hitting you over the head with in this book.)

HIT increases the metabolic rate after exercise and burns more calories during it than cardio, which is likely one reason it's more effective for fat loss. In a study published in the International Journal of Obesity[97], a number of young women was divided into two groups, one performing HIT, and the other doing steady-state aerobic exercise. (There was also a control group that did nothing.)

Both groups showed similar increases in cardiorespiratory fitness.

But despite exercising less than half the time as the aerobic exercisers, *the HIT group lost over 11% of their body fat, and the aerobic group lost none.* This agrees with other results that show aerobic exercise next to useless for fat loss. Furthermore, the HIT exercisers gained about 0.1 kg of lean mass and the aerobic group lost 0.9 kg of lean mass, although the researchers considered this result to be not statistically significant. Nevertheless, it agrees with other studies that show aerobic exercisers losing lean body mass.

Another important result was that the HIT exercisers dropped their fasting insulin levels by 31%, whereas the steady-state aerobic group lowered theirs by only 9%. The extent to which each individual decreased her fasting insulin levels was highly correlated to the amount of fat lost; that is, the more fat lost, the greater the decrease in fasting insulin.

The insulin results are incredibly important, since they show the power of HIT to improve metabolic function, and thus can be a potent weapon in fighting diabetes and the metabolic syndrome. Generally, you want fasting insulin to be as low as possible — though no lower — and fasting insulin is tightly correlated with good metabolic control, and with good health overall.

Rightly suspecting that HIT would have beneficial effects for diabetics, some researchers took a group of diabetics and had them do HIT for 12 weeks.[98] The diabetics reduced their HbA1c, a measure of blood sugar control (lower is better), and reduced the amount of fat in their liver by a whopping 39%. They also improved the structure and function of their heart.

Keep in mind that all of the results I've mentioned so far were due solely to HIT; there was no dietary component, and the participants ate what they usually did. Adding a healthy diet, low in sugar and refined carbohydrates, to a high-intensity training protocol would give even better results in terms of fat loss and glucose control.

HIT, as we've just seen, can be a safe exercise mode for ill people, as with the diabetics. It's been used effectively in people with diabetes, heart failure, and in those who have has heart attacks. (Needless to say, any exercise prescription should be cleared with your doctor, and that goes double if you have any kind of illness.)

No more time excuses

Back when I used to run long distances, I would often get up an hour earlier in the morning when I wanted to get in a good training run before work. All told, during the course of a week, my running took up probably 6 to 8 hours of my time, considering warming up, cooling down, extra long runs, etc. Running is a time-consuming form of exercise, as are many others.

The mainstream fitness establishment for decades now has extolled steady-state aerobic exercise done at a relatively low intensity, saying that it is uniquely suited for cardiorespiratory fitness. As we've seen from numerous studies and examples in this book, that, like so many other things the fitness folks have been telling us, just isn't true. Not that aerobic exercise doesn't contribute to better health and fitness – it does. But other exercises, like HIT and strength training, do this also, and do it better, and help you in other ways, such as fat loss and muscle strength, as well.

One result of the fitness people telling us this is a paradoxical decrease in the amount of exercise people could potentially do. The most-cited reason people give is lack of time. They figure that if they don't have 45 minutes to an hour a day to devote to exercise, then they're just not going to bother.

So the idea of HIT training is liberating and has the potential to get many more people to exercise, since you can do it, including rest intervals, in 30 minutes a *week*. One can also easily design a strength training program that has very similar length of time. (Of course, if you want to be a bodybuilder you'll need more time than that, but most people can benefit greatly with only 30 to 60 minutes a week of strength training.)

When doctors prescribe exercise to patients, their long-term adherence to exercise programs is abysmal; sometimes less than 50% of people remain in an exercise program at the end of six months. Very likely the reasons for this are time and boredom. HIT can overcome this hurdle.

Keep that in mind: next time you're tempted to excuse yourself from exercise because of lack of time, remember HIT, and go do some.

A word of warning about HIT: the intensity of the exercise is much greater than what you're normally used to, and this can be off-putting for some people. The upside is that the intensity is short-lasting. When you start, you don't need to go for the all-out intensity of the Wingate test; just do what you're capable of, and increase the intensity of your sessions as you are able. The important thing is to do it.

I've added HIT to my exercise program, as it makes an ideal counterpart to strength training. I'm in the gym once every three days lifting weights, and once every three days I do a HIT routine that takes me about ten minutes. And once every three days I take it easy and go for a walk. It's a good, sustainable exercise program for me, one that doesn't tax my body so much that I need days to recover. Sustainability and recovery are very important; I've seen guys—and a few gals—on exercise regimes that leave them feeling pretty lousy most of the time due to extreme fatigue. Don't do that to yourself, as it not only feels bad, but it's bad for your health.

High-intensity training routines

The original high-intensity routine was the Tabata workout, which consists of 20 seconds of all-out effort on a stationary cycle, punctuated by 10 second rest intervals, done for a total of 4 minutes. That's 8 all-out intervals.

The Tabata routine can be adapted to other types of exercises as well as time lengths. For instance, here's a Tabata workout that last 20 minutes and is done with calisthenics. Each exercise is done twice, and there's a one-minute rest interval between segments.[99]

	Minute 1	Minute 2	Minute 3	Minute 4
Seg 1	High Knee Run	Plank Punch	Jump Jacks	Side Skaters
Seg 2	Jump Rope	In/Out Boat	Line Jumps	Push-Ups
Seg 3	Burpees	Russian Twists	Squats	Lunges
Seg 4	Mt. Climber	Push-Ups	Split Squat	Box Jumps

Or, you could take any exercise singly or in combination with another and do the entire workout based on that. For example, do a Tabata workout with burpees only, 20 seconds of burpees, 10 seconds rest, for 4 minutes. In a short amount of time, you'll have done a tremendous amount of exercise. In fact, when you first try it, you may not be able to complete it. Burpees are tough. Or alternate burpees with push-ups and jumping jacks. You get the idea, I'm sure.

Beyond the Tabata workout, different time intervals could be used, and that's probably a better place to start. Use a rest interval long enough to recover your normal breathing before going to the next set. One variation I often use is a combination of jump rope, push-ups, and air squats. I'll jump rope for about one minute, rest for perhaps 30 seconds, then do push-ups for 30 seconds, rest again, then on to the next one. It looks like this:

1. Jump rope, 60 seconds
2. Rest 30 seconds
3. Push-ups, 30 seconds
4. Rest 30 seconds to one minute
5. Jump rope, 60 seconds, alternatively, jumping jacks
6. Rest 30 to 60 seconds
7. Air squats, 30 seconds
8. Rest 30 to 60 seconds
9. Etc.

Do this for a total of 8 intervals. This gives you a great, whole-body workout. In case you're wondering about how to time this, some folks who do HIT use a timer, and there are special HIT timers available. I do not. I count my jump rope reps in my head – about 120 reps is good for one minute, more or less. I also count push-ups and other calisthenics to give myself a rough idea of the amount of time spent.

The exact timing isn't critical, because as you can see, the workouts themselves vary tremendously in timing, number of intervals, rest periods, and types of exercise.

When you first start, HIT will take some getting used to. It is much more intense than a steady-state aerobic exercise. It will feel uncomfortable. Get into it gradually and don't let the fact that you are relatively untrained stop you from performing HIT and making progress in it.

Rest days are extremely important. You don't want to do this daily, as you need recovery days when your body builds strength and endurance. If you're relatively out of shape, a couple of times a week ought to be plenty.

If you do any strength training, adding a HIT session once a week may be more than enough. Unfortunately, there's only so much direction one can give in a book, because people are of different ages, weights, and fitness levels, so you will have to be in charge of setting the level of your personal HIT program.

In the gym

HIT can be done nicely in the gym with weights. The key here is to use lighter weights or even just body weight. In weightlifting, good form is required in order to lessen the chance of injuries; when you're moving fast, as in HIT, you don't want to be throwing around heavy weights for that reason.

Here's a sample program, one that I've used, for an in-gym HIT routine.

- Stationary cycle, all-out 20 to 30 seconds
- Rest up to one minute
- Dips, fast pace, 30 seconds
- Rest
- Pull-ups, fast pace, 30 seconds
- Rest
- Barbell curls, lighter weight, fast pace, 30 seconds
- Rest

Repeat for two bouts, giving a total of 8 intervals. You'll know you've had a workout with this one.

If your gym has the right equipment, you can do things like a farmer's walk (walking with heavy weights in both hands) or sled-pushing.

It bears repeating that these are very intense workouts. Do not do them every day, and if you also strength train, once a week may suffice. Ease into your Tabata or other HIT routine slowly.

10-20-30 training, and 10-training

A form of HIT was invented to overcome one of the biggest objections to this type of exercise: its intensity. Some people find it too taxing, and then stop doing it.

In 10-20-30 training (note that 30-20-10 is more accurate, but doesn't have quite the same ring to it), the exerciser works out at a relaxed pace for 30 seconds, goes to a moderate pace for 20 seconds, and then goes all out for 10 seconds. Each one is a set, and each set can be repeated five or six times.

Most people seem to find this much easier to take than some of the HIT regimens previously described. The question is, does it work?

It does work, indeed.[100] In a group of already trained recreational runners, 10-20-30 training increased cardiorespiratory fitness and lowered blood pressure, and substantially lowered the time to run 5 kilometers, compared to the group that continued to perform steady-state exercise—jogging, in this case.

Once again, the superiority of HIT to aerobics is demonstrated. What's more, you can perform this workout in six minutes.

The question arises as to whether the relaxed and moderate paced segments of this routine are even necessary. The actual high-intensity part is only 10 seconds of the total, and this part is what causes physiological adaptations. My sense of this matter is that the other segments could be dispensed with.

So, for example, you can sprint all out for 10 seconds, then walk back to your starting point, then do it again. I've done a workout just like this. (I find that when I do several 20 to 30 second all-out sprints, I feel like I need days to recover properly. Not so with this method.) Let's call this form of HIT "10-training".

It can be adapted to different types of exercise: rowing machine, stationary cycle or bicycle, calisthenics. To my mind this makes an ideal form for beginners, and may be all anyone needs to improve cardiorespiratory fitness. Ideally, for this type of HIT as for others, you should choose an exercise or exercises that work the entire musculature, i.e. don't do sprints or stationary bike only. Choose some calisthenics, or light dumbbells, do push-ups, etc.

Takeaway points

- High-intensity training is a more efficient way to train than aerobics
- HIT has many of the same benefits as strength training
- HIT is much better than aerobics for fat loss, lean gains, and improvement in insulin sensitivity and metabolic health
- HIT eliminates the time excuse for exercise
- There are many forms of HIT, and it's easy to design your own workout
- HIT requires plenty of rest and recovery; do not do it daily
- HIT variations, such as 10-20-30 and 10-training, may be as effective but less difficult

Chapter 9: How to implement a basic strength-training program

One of the biggest roadblocks for anyone contemplating starting a strength-training routine is lack of knowledge as to where to begin. Some people think that it's just too complicated, requires some kind of insider knowledge, and that if not done right it's better not done at all. There's just enough truth to these suppositions to stop people from doing it, but in reality, you can learn how to do it in very little time, and with a little practice, the techniques will come easy.

A further barrier is psychological, and it has to do with some of the guys in the gym, in bodybuilding parlance, the bros. In any gym, there are going to be some standout bodybuilders, big guys who lift heavy weights, grunt and groan while doing so, who drop their weights with a loud crash, and who sometimes look intimidating, at least to "normal" people.

In reality, most of these guys are friendly and welcoming. They're happy to see new faces in the weight room, and if you need help or advice, are usually more than willing to lend a hand. So don't let them stop you from getting in there, mixing it up with them, and lifting weights.

Most of the people doing strength training are not bros, however, they're ordinary people.

With that out of the way, let's look at the rationale and the practice of a basic strength-training program.

How muscles grow

Muscle tissue is "plastic", that is, it responds to environmental influence or the lack of it, and grows, metabolizes, or shrinks according to the kind and amount of stimulus applied to it. In strength training, we load weight on the muscle and move it through a range of movement, thus applying a stress to it. The muscle responds to the stimulus by increasing or decreasing various biochemical and physiological mechanisms that will cause it to grow.

In a state of nature, humans need to respond to a stimulus like this by getting stronger, as it is a matter of survival to do so.

By applying this stimulus on a regular basis, and increasing it, muscles get both stronger and larger. Muscle growth is referred to as "hypertrophy".

Lifting a weight, or maneuvering the levers of a weight machine, for one movement, up and down, or back and forth as the case may be, is a "repetition", commonly known as a "rep". A group of reps done together is a "set".

Generally, more reps and/or heavier weights cause greater muscular growth. Lifting a very heavy weight that you can only manage for one rep does not cause much muscular growth, since the stimulus for growth is one of weight multiplied by time under tension or repetitions completed. So when you perform an exercise, you will be doing so with a weight that you can lift or move for between 8 and 12 reps, which gives the best anabolic (growth) stimulus. More reps than 12 has more of a cardiorespiratory component than it does a strength training component, and fewer reps with heavier weights more of a pure strength component.

Compound exercises

Compound exercises are those in which the movement of the weight or machine requires two or more joints. A simple example is a squat, or you can just think of it as a deep knee bend. When you squat down, you use the joints at the knees and at the hips, so this is a compound exercise. A proper strength training program, that is, one that will improve both strength and muscle size on the one hand, and metabolic and cardiorespiratory health on the other, will consist mainly of compound exercises. These are the ones you want to do.

A non-compound exercise, sometimes referred to as an isolation exercise, requires only one joint for movement. An example is the biceps curl, in which a weight is lifted by one or both arms; the arms start fully extended in a downward position, and the weight is lifted to the shoulder, with the biceps muscle in the upper arm doing most of the work. While this type of exercise will cause the exercised muscle to grow, it is relatively ineffective for getting the health effects we want from strength training. As you get stronger and more experienced, you may want to incorporate a few of these exercises into your routine, but at the beginning, you should concentrate on compound exercises, getting them right, and becoming stronger overall, not in growing isolated muscles.

The main compound exercises are all that you need to do for a good, whole-body strength training routine. Further along in your training, as you become more adept at lifting weights, you can explore variations on these exercises, of which a nearly infinite variety exist. If you're just starting a strength training program, you should learn these basic compound exercises, and your routine should consist mainly of them.

There are five main compound exercises, six if you add deadlifts.

Squat and leg press. Traditional squats are done with a barbell supported at the top of the back at shoulder level, and then the person squats down at least parallel to the knees, and gets back up again. There's a definite technique involved here, and beginners or even most people can use a leg press machine, which doesn't require as much skill to use. Squats have some advantages over leg presses in terms of applying a stimulus to more muscles.

Squat technique is not difficult to learn, and you can start by using an unloaded Olympic barbell, which weighs 45 pounds. If you can't handle that much weight, just do repeated squats with no weights until you build up your strength. Or grab a couple of light dumbbells, one in each hand, and squat with them.

Before you use heavier weight in the squat, be sure you have good technique.

The leg press involves the person in a sitting position with his or her legs bent and pressed against a plate, which in turn is weighted. The person then pushes on the plate, extending the legs to a straight position, and then moves the legs back to the original position.

Both of these exercises work the thigh muscles ("quads") as well as the gluteal muscles ("glutes", the buttocks), although the squats apply more stimulus to the glutes than does the leg press. Many people (including myself) incorporate both of these exercises into their routines. I've found that I require the leg press for maximal stimulation of my quads.

Shoulder press: This exercise works the shoulder muscles ("deltoids" or "delts"), and entails raising a weight starting from the shoulders, with arms bent, extending the arms overhead into a straight position, and then back down. This move can be done with either free weights or a machine, and can also be done sitting down.

Just as in the squat, if you can't manage a lot of weight in this move in the beginning, you can use an unloaded barbell or a pair of lighter dumbbells. Or use a machine set at a light weight.

The muscles of the shoulder are relatively small compared to, say, those in the chest, and therefore the weight you use in the shoulder press will generally be quite a bit less than for some other upper body exercises.

Bench or chest press: This exercise works the chest muscles ("pecs") and to a lesser extent the shoulders and the triceps (muscles on the back of the upper arm). In a bench press, the user lies flat on a bench, with a weighted barbell in a rack above and slightly behind him. He then removes the weight from the rack, lowers it to chest height, and then pushes it back up again. A chest press is a machine move that accomplishes nearly the same thing, often with the user in an upright, seated position, who then pushes the weight forward and then allows it to come back.

Bench presses have the disadvantage that with heavier weights, the user should have a "spot", which is a person who stands behind him and assists him if necessary, normally on just the last rep. A spot is often necessary because if the user can't push the weight back up, say after several reps, he then has a weighted barbell that he can't move stuck on top of his chest. Needless to say, that's an uncomfortable and possibly even dangerous position to be in, and it's happened to me. I've mostly used a chest press machine ever since.

Most people who aren't attempting to become the next Mr. Universe will do fine sticking to a chest press machine, or if you insist on doing a bench press, make sure you can handle it and start with a light weight, and/or have someone spot you. Another safe alternative to the bench press using a barbell is to use dumbbells. In the dumbbell press, one usually grasps the dumbbells before reclining on either a flat or an inclined bench, then presses the dumbbells for a set, after which the weights can be dropped. No danger of getting stuck underneath them.

The chest muscles are capable of becoming quite large, and the bench press and its variations play a large role in the workouts of serious bodybuilders.

Rows: This exercise comes in a number of different flavors, but in essence it consists of pulling a weight toward the body. It works muscles in the back and the arms.

Bent-over rows consists of grasping a weighted barbell, bending the waist at about a 45 degree angle, and pulling the weight up to just below chest level, then relaxing back into the starting position. There are also T-bar rows, consisting of pulling up the end of a barbell from the floor, or using a special device for this. As with the other exercises, rows can be done on machines, one such being a seated cable row: in a sitting position, you pull a cable attached to a weight. These are arguably safer for the back than using a barbell.

Pull-ups, chin-ups, and pull-downs: Pull-ups are a familiar exercise, and consist of grasping an overhead bar with palms facing away from you, pulling yourself up so that your chin is level with it, and then letting yourself down. Chin-ups are the same exercise, but with palms facing toward you. Pull-downs are done on a machine, and this involves pulling a weighted bar down to chest level, then letting it back up. All of these exercises work muscles in the arms ("biceps") and at the side of the back ("lats").

Pull-ups, despite being a free form exercise, are generally safe even for beginners, but unfortunately most beginners don't have the strength to pull up their entire body weight, so they won't be able to do even one. (Chin-ups are somewhat easier for most people.) That's where the pull-downs come in, since you can set the weight at well below body weight if that's what you need. There are also machines on which the user stands on a platform that is counter-weighted, and does pull-ups with less than entire body weight.

Deadlift: This exercise consists of bending/squatting and grasping a weighted barbell, then straightening the legs and back and lifting the barbell to just below the hips, with arms straight. Basically, this move is just picking a weight up off the floor, and setting it back down again. The deadlift works muscles in the legs, buttocks, and back.

This is my favorite exercise; there's nothing like being able to deadlift 300 pounds, and it feels like quite the accomplishment. (Many experienced weightlifters deadlift far more than that.)

On the other hand, the deadlift must be done with excellent form or you risk injury, and most regular people who work out in the gym never perform this exercise due to a fear that they may hurt their back, a fear that's not wholly unfounded. I know of no machines that duplicate this movement. Some gyms may have a type of barbell known as a trap bar, which makes it easier to use correct form in the deadlift. If you decide to give the deadlift a go, start with light weight, and get some instruction from an experienced trainer. Most young, healthy people who want to add serious amounts of muscle should learn this move and incorporate it into their routine; otherwise, if you're a beginner and/or not enthusiastic about the deadlift, it may be omitted from your routine. That being said, even the old ladies with osteoporosis that I discussed in another chapter were doing deadlifts, some even lifting the equivalent of their own body weight.

This is a good place to emphasize that not all or even most people who work in a gym are experienced trainers, especially if you go to some outfit like Planet Fitness. No offense to them — the employees, not Planet Fitness — but many are just attendants, so asking one of these people the proper form for the deadlift or any other exercise may be asking for trouble.

Free weights vs machines

Many guys (and a few gals) who are serious about strength training insist that free weights, that is barbells and dumbbells, are much better for training and muscular development. Use of free weights also better promotes neurological conditioning, that is, the connection and coordination between the nervous and skeletal muscle systems.

While free weights generally have greater efficacy in building muscle, machines certainly have their place, and not just for beginning strength trainers either.

The premise of this book is that almost everyone who is able to strength train will benefit from it, and that includes girls, young women, little old ladies and little old men, the obese, the skinny, and the weak. For all of these people, machines offer a good option for starting a strength training program. Machines simply require less skill and training, and offer much better protection from injury than do free weights.

I think that trying to get an older person or someone who is recovering from illness or injury to strength train by showing them the proper form for doing a squat, for example, may be counterproductive. This may needlessly complicate things and may stop some people from taking up strength training.

I want to encourage strength training for everyone by making the process as uncomplicated as possible, and stating that you must use free weights and complicated movements that require lots of instruction may intimidate some people. I believe that you should get into the gym, for sure there will be a bit of learning to do, but it need not be complicated.

Myself, I use both free weights and machines, as needed. Most healthy, young to middle-aged men who aim to pack on large amounts of muscle use free weights, at least in part like me. That is more than fine, but if you just want an increase in muscle strength and a good conditioning routine, machines offer an entirely acceptable alternative.

Warming up

As with almost any exercise of greater intensity than mere walking, you should warm up before beginning a strength training session. The warm-up need not be long or complicated, but doing it will help protect against pulled muscles and some other injuries.

Stretching: I spend a grand total of about 30 seconds in stretching before I begin my workout. I touch my toes a few times gently and easily to stretch hamstrings. Then I stand up straight with arms extended upward as high as they will go. Next, I lean against a wall at about a 70 degree angle and press against it, so that back, hamstrings, and calves are stretched. That's about it. Too much stretching can have a detrimental effect on muscle power, so I don't recommend extensive stretching; it's not necessary and could hurt strength training performance. This isn't yoga.

Warm-up: Before beginning an individual strength training exercise such as a compound lift, go through the motions of the lift with very light weight. For example, on the day I work the back, I start with the deadlift. I grab an unloaded Olympic bar, which weighs 45 pounds (~20 kg), and perform 10 repetitions with it. Next, I add two large plates to it, so that the total weight is 135 pounds (~60 kg), and perform another 10 repetitions. After this, I feel fully warmed up and add as much as weight as necessary to do my main lifts.

When you move to the next exercise, warm up for that one too. If you've been exercising heavily already, that may not take much, but there may be muscles that haven't been used much up to that point in your session, so warm them up. In a shoulder press, use an unloaded bar for a warm-up set, or set your machine to a light weight. Follow the same principle for all your lifts: at least one and maybe two sets at light weight before you lift heavy.

Should you exercise to failure?

As noted above, one complete motion with a weight or on a machine is said to be a "rep", and several reps in a group, usually of 8 to 12 but it can be any number, is a "set".

Most physical trainers and coaches advocate lifting a weight to "failure", which means that you perform repetitions of the motion until you literally can't do anymore, a state called voluntary failure, because the muscles involved are spent. Normally one will then rest for one minute up to several minutes, and do the same set again, to failure.

A fair amount of academic research supports the idea that lifting to failure is optimal for muscle growth, that is, it provides the greatest stimulus. If you don't lift to failure, the muscle isn't getting enough of the signals needed for it to grow, so the thinking goes, because anything less than failure means that the muscles are working within a capacity they already have.

Some trainers advocate lifting to failure only on the last set, since many people find it both mentally and physically too taxing.

Personally, I follow the first prescription and on virtually every set, I lift to failure.

Is it necessary for the average person who wants to start a strength training program to lift to failure? No, it is not.

Every repetition of a weightlifting movement provides a stimulus for the growth of muscle. Since we're not all college athletes or wannabe Arnolds, most of us don't need to have the absolute maximal or optimal stimulus for muscle growth, especially at first. What I'm saying here is that the issue of lifting to failure is similar to the free weights versus machines issue. Asking the average person who just wants a good conditioning workout to lift to failure may be asking too much.

Most people who are not used to high-level athletics may not realize the intensity involved in lifting to failure.

By all means, if you're healthy and strong and really want to pack on muscle, lift to failure. But if you're not in that category, I wouldn't worry about it.

Number of sets

How many sets of each exercise should you do? Let's say you can do 8 reps of leg presses using 150 pounds on the machine. You do them, rest for a minute or three, then do 8 more reps. Do you rest some more, do another set and just keep going?

Those new to strength training may be surprised to learn that the number of sets one should perform to maximize muscle growth is controversial. Without going too deep into the details, some academic studies have found that one set of an exercise maximizes the stimulus for muscle growth, and that doing more sets does not increase that stimulus. Other studies have found that up to 8 sets can increase the stimulus and thus increase muscle growth.

How are we to make sense of this, and does it matter for the average person who wants to strength train?

There are knowledgeable people who advocate training with only one set, so long as it's to failure. There are other equally knowledgeable people who advocate doing many sets. A program called German volume training, for instance, calls for up to 10 sets of each exercise.

The older, classic bodybuilding routines usually called for 3 sets of 10 reps for each exercise or muscle group. For the average person, that's a good place to start. Performing 3 sets gives you practice doing the exercise; the first set also can serve as a warmup for the next two sets. You can do all the sets for the same exercise in a row, together, and this is the pattern many bodybuilders follow. For general conditioning, you can mix up the sets for different exercises and muscle groups; this is known as circuit training.

If you do more sets, you at least have the possibility of stimulating more muscle growth than if you perform fewer sets. So why wouldn't you do more sets, all other things being equal? The problem with just doing lots of sets, or just generally working out harder and longer, lies in a very important concept in strength training, *recovery*.

Recovery

When you train muscles by lifting weights or through other forms of strength training, you place a stress on them. This stress actually causes muscles to break down, and when they have time to rest and recover, the muscles build themselves back up again, stronger than before.

However, muscles don't recover from a hard workout in hours, or even a day. Usually it takes several days and maybe even up to one week before full recovery. Before that full recovery, muscles are weaker than they were before the workout and before they were stressed.

Recovery is a very important but, alas, sadly neglected component of strength training. Muscles do not grow in the gym; on the contrary, the gym is where muscles are broken down. Muscles grow when they are resting. Doing more and more exercise, in this case more sets, does not necessarily mean that you will get more or faster muscle growth, since more exercise requires more recovery time. If not, we could just spend every day in the gym and get ripped. Obviously, most of us can't do that. We'd be wiped out and feel extremely fatigued all the time.

What's more, when you are fatigued and train for strength, you won't be able to give muscles the optimal workout in terms of weight, reps, or sets, leading to a suboptimal workout.

This brings us back to the question of how many sets of each exercise you should perform, and how many times a week you should train.

The more sets you do, and the more frequently you do them, the longer the time you will need for recovery. Young, healthy people need less time for recovery than older people, and variation of the amount of recovery time needed between individuals is high.

Many young people, especially men, get very gung-ho about bodybuilding and try to get into the gym four or five times a week, or even daily. For them, this can work for awhile, but it can lead to the physiological state known as overtraining.

In overtraining, constant fatigue is a prominent symptom, and upper respiratory infections such as colds and flu can become more frequent. Of course, strength training doesn't have a monopoly on overtraining; it's often seen among runners and in other sports, most commonly in elite athletes or simply those who push themselves too much. *Overtraining is an unhealthy condition to be in.*

The amount of recovery time people need varies greatly, and depends on:

- frequency of strength training sessions
- the intensity and duration of those sessions
- age
- sex
- degree of fitness
- quantity and quality of food
- quantity and quality of sleep
- amount of time spent at a physically demanding job vs at home
- genetic background

So it's impossible to lay down hard-and-fast commandments for the amount of rest and recovery time needed for any given individual.

Most of you reading this who decide to start a strength training program will be doing a whole-body workout. (As opposed to a split workout, discussed below.) A good rule of thumb for those doing whole-body routines is: *do not train for strength daily*. Take a minimum of one rest day between gym sessions.

You must, to use a cliché, listen to your body. If you feel fatigued, taking a rest day is better than trying to hammer out a gym session. My own workout schedule is once every three days; I find that if I try to train more often than that, I'm very tired on rest days, and I can't give it my best in the gym on workout days. This last item is important: if you find that you're not able to do as much in terms of weight lifted or number of reps and sets as you were able to do the last time you worked out, then *you need more rest*. It's better to walk out of the gym at that point rather than to continue a suboptimal workout that will leave you more fatigued than before.

A somewhat more objective method for determining whether you've overtrained is to check your heart rate when resting in bed before getting up in the morning. If your heart rate is 10 or more beats per minute higher than it normally is, you're overtraining and need more rest. Go back to bed. (If you're heart rate isn't that elevated over baseline, it doesn't necessarily mean that you're not overtraining though.)

A few things that may help you have a quicker recovery time include:

- more dietary protein
- adequate hydration
- saunas
- easy walking days

Sometimes you hear physical trainers and coaches and other people who should know better saying things like "there's no such thing as overtraining, you're just a wimp". Or, "even if you don't feel your best, go lift some heavy weights anyway". My advice: ignore them. They're wrong.

Some strength training writers advocate once a week training only. On the other hand, bodybuilding magazines and websites often claim that if you're not in the gym almost daily, you won't make any strength or fitness gains. The middle ground is two to three training sessions a week.

For those who want to improve their muscular strength and metabolic health without necessarily striving for large amounts of muscular growth, a once a week session may be enough, provided that workout is intense enough. This also assumes that other types of exercise are done on most off-gym days, i.e. that you're not completely sedentary outside of the gym.

Most people will, I believe, fall into the category of needing strength training two to three days a week. This will be enough to build strength and fitness without overtraining. I believe that the vast majority of people should train for strength no more than three times a week.

How long should you spend in the gym each time you train? Again, this varies a great deal depending on the individual, but for most people, one hour at a time is plenty, and it's possible to get in a decent workout in half that time. For most people, one hour should suffice, and more than that can make for longer recovery time and possibly lead to overtraining if done often enough.

The take-home lesson is that more sets and more training days do not necessarily lead to a better training outcome, i.e. greater muscular strength and better cardiometabolic health.

Split routines

Muscles can require several days or even up to a week to completely recover from the stress placed on them during strength training. In addition, if someone who trains wants to do multiple sets and exercises for each muscle group, then a gym session of perhaps one hour doesn't leave adequate time to train the whole body. Put these two factors together and you come up with the concept of split routines.

Split routines mean that you don't work out the whole body each time you train. For example, a two-way split may have you training the back, chest, and arms on one day, and the next session you train legs, shoulders, and abs. (This is in fact the schedule I use.) Another common split schedule is to train lower body and upper body on alternate days. Some dedicated bodybuilders will even use four-way splits.

Split routines allow you to work much harder on any given muscle group. If, say, you want to work out the chest with three sets of chest press, three sets of cable crossovers, and three sets of dumbbell flies, then your chest muscles are going to need a good, long rest afterward and won't be ready for another workout for quite awhile. With a split routine, you won't train the same muscles until a week or more has gone by, allowing them plenty of time for rest and recovery.

If you train intensely and more often than twice a week, with a goal of large gains in muscle growth, a split routine is probably the way to go. They're not necessary if you train with less intensity, less often, and/or with the goal of general conditioning.

Taking some time off from the gym can often be helpful too. If every six to eight weeks you skip a week for rest, that can actually help your gains by keeping you fresh and rested. You will experience little to no loss of muscle by taking a week off from the gym. The same applies if you need more recovery time: just skip the next scheduled gym session and you'll be better off than if you force yourself to go when you're too fatigued.

Don't skip leg day

This section won't apply to all of you, but there's a common type of person seen in the gym, usually a young man who wants to make himself look more manly. He trains his upper body intensely, but never trains his legs. Maybe he figures that no one will notice.

The result can be humorous: a man with well-built chest, arms, and shoulders, and stick-thin legs.

Even if you don't care about the aesthetics of skinny legs and a wildly asymmetric body, you should keep in mind that the lower body – legs and buttocks – contain more than half of all your skeletal muscle. For good physical conditioning and health, you must also train your lower body.

What does training the lower body look like? Well, not everyone will want to do heavy squats, but the leg press is a good substitute. However, beware of machines that promise to train the legs but provide only a simple (not compound) exercise. Examples of these are leg extensions and leg curls. I'm not saying you can't do these in addition to squats or leg press, but they don't provide enough of a workout for the legs on their own.

Then there's that funny machine that only women seem to use, the one that has them spreading and closing their legs. It looks rather peculiar, and it's also just a lousy leg exercise. Ladies (and girls), stay off that machine and do your squats or leg presses, which will give you much better results in terms of both appearance and health.

Which brings us to the next topic.

Strength training for women

Historically only men have trained for strength, but that's changed a lot in recent years, and more women are doing it. Are there any special considerations in strength training for women?

Only a few, really. Women should strength train with the same intensity as men do. The type of exercises chosen may vary somewhat.

Many women believe that because they're not trying to become big and muscular, that their workouts should be different, for instance, that they should use lighter weights or work out less often. The main difference between men's and women's attitudes and ideas about strength training is that most women don't think that they need to do it at all. The real difference is in exercise selection.

Those women who do want to strength train often have a funny idea about something called "toning". They'll just lift some light weights for the appropriate body part, and they believe that will improve their appearance. Two common examples of this are the leg spreading contraption I mentioned above, and working on the triceps (back of the upper arm) with a very light weight.

Toning is a myth. If you want muscles to be firm and strong, they should receive solid training, not a quick, sloppily done set that will do next to nothing for them.

Sagging triceps are an unfortunate sign of aging that's often more prominent in women than in men, and naturally women would like to be rid of them. Sagging body parts like the triceps are usually due to a lack of strong muscle combined with an excess of fat. The solution to sagging arms isn't toning, it's a decent, whole-body strength training program. This will strengthen and grow sagging muscles as well as aid in fat loss.

Toning is not the only myth for women in strength training. Another common misconception many women have is that, if they work out like men, they will end up with the muscular physique of men, which hardly any women want, understandably.

The answer to that myth is that 99% of women couldn't attain a masculine, muscular body if they wanted to. Building large, noticeable amounts of muscle is difficult even for men, and all the more so for women. It requires dedication, time, hard training, and... something else.

That something else, an important factor in muscle growth, is the hormone testosterone, and while women have some testosterone, men have about ten times as much. Without testosterone, anyone will have great difficulty in building visible muscle, whether they're female or male. In fact, large doses of testosterone given to men cause muscle growth *even without exercise of any kind*.

Another reason women won't and can't develop a masculine physique is that women have higher amounts of body fat than men do. Whereas a man may be considered "fit" if his body fat percentage is in the range of 14 to

17%, for a woman the same numbers are 21 to 24%.[101] Even female athletes have more body fat than do male athletes. This is normal and natural, as women have the ability to bear children, and pregnancy and nursing require the greater energy stores that come with more body fat; women can in fact become infertile if their body fat drops too low. Much of the body fat in both women and men is subcutaneous, that is, beneath the skin.

More subcutaneous body fat means that muscles just don't show as much, since they're covered by a layer of fat. Men with greater than normal amounts of fat don't show a lot of muscle either; that's why bodybuilders are so concerned with having low body fat.

What about female bodybuilders who have large, well-defined muscles and low levels of body fat, i.e. they are, to use bodybuilding lingo, "ripped"? Well, for one thing, they are very dedicated to their sport, and have training and dieting regimens that tend to the extreme. Some of them also take anabolic steroids, which are testosterone-like drugs that cause muscle growth and fat loss, leading to the "ripped" look. The ultra-low body fat of female bodybuilders is not a very healthy thing to have, whether brought on by steroids or not.

So, women should have no fears about overdoing it at the gym. Women should perhaps place more emphasis on the lower body – legs and glutes – less on the upper body. The same considerations for number of sets and frequency of training apply to women as they do to men. Naturally, most women will be training with lighter weights than most men do, since women are generally smaller than men and have less natural muscular strength, but when they train, they should train with intensity.

Aside from the fact that both sexes can develop sarcopenia (muscle-wasting) as they age, many women who don't have full-blown sarcopenia still lose muscle and don't look as attractive as they could.

It's not uncommon to see somewhat older women, let's say in their 50s and 60s, who have kept or recovered their slender figures. Many of them have worked hard with diet and aerobic exercise to do so. But by the time they're that age they've lost a fairly large amount of muscle, and instead of slender with nice curves, have more of a stick-figure look, basically just skin and bones. Probably most of these women have never given a second or even a first thought to muscle loss and how it makes them look, but they should. A strength training program for women like this can make them look more attractive in addition to making them healthier.

Form and tempo

Weights should be lifted with good form for two reasons: one, to get the best muscle-growth stimulus possible for the amount of work that you put in, and two, to avoid hurting yourself. These considerations are less important in the use of exercise machines, since they take form out of the equation to a certain extent. If you're injured, you can't train, so taking the time to ensure that you understand and use good form saves you a lot of trouble over the long run.

The proper form to use differs for each exercise and is unfortunately beyond the scope of this book, as a thorough explanation of each exercise would require a separate training manual. Probably the easiest way to learn the proper form of an exercise is to watch an instructional video on it, many of which can be found on YouTube. Another way is to get some instruction from a trainer at your gym first, although you should be sure that this gym person really knows how to train. I don't want to give the impression that proper form is difficult either to learn or to perform, but you should have some basic knowledge first to make sure that you have a safe workout. Otherwise, the use of exercise machines is perfectly fine.

I also don't want to give the impression that strength training is especially prone to injuring people, because it is not. It is generally a safe form of exercise, and is vastly safer than sports like football and mountain biking, and even quite a bit safer than distance running.[102] Bodybuilding has an injury rate of between 0.24 and 1.00 injuries per 1000 hours of training, compared to endurance sports like distance running at 1.4 to 5.4 injuries per 1000 hours. (Other forms of strength training, such as power and Olympic lifting, have higher injury rates than bodybuilding, but these types of training require special skills and are for elite athletes only. In this book, strength training refers to a bodybuilding type of program.)

But as in other sports, it is possible to pull muscles, injure the back, and so on, and a little knowledge can go a long way keeping you injury-free.

If you're lifting a weight and something hurts, *stop*. While strength training often causes discomfort, pain is another matter and is a sign that you're injuring yourself.

As for muscle stimulus and form, the most common mistake that leads to a poor stimulus, and to injuries as well, is throwing weights around. Some people like to use weights heavier than they can move through a proper motion, and when they do this, they then leverage their entire body to move the weight. Don't do this. Use a weight light enough that you can move properly.

The law of reversibility in strength training states that one should be able to reverse the trajectory of the weight and its motion at any time in the course of a lift. If you cannot do this, the most likely cause is the use of an inappropriately heavy weight.

It can be tempting when in the gym to show off with the heavy weight that one is lifting, but this is a good way to injure yourself. Keep in mind also that heavier isn't necessarily better. A few more reps rather than heavier weight may give you more stimulus for muscle growth while lessening your chance of injury.

Exercise machines, as I noted, make proper form easier, and I think that most beginners, and even many people who are not, would do just fine by sticking to them, as they can provide a good cardiorespiratory and metabolic workout. After you get stronger and more experienced, you can learn the barbell and dumbbell moves. In the strength training world you'll come across diametrically opposed opinions if you read more in this area, but not everyone who wants to train for strength is a young, healthy man whose goal is to pack on lots of muscle.

Tempo is the pace at which you move the weight through its proper motion, and this applies to both free weights and machines. Muscle grows through a stimulus, and that stimulus depends on time under tension, that is, the amount of weight being moved and the time taken to do that. For example, taking one minute to move a 30 pound weight in one set (in any exercise) provides more stimulus than moving a 20 pound weight the same length of time; moving any weight for one minute also provides more stimulus than moving the same weight for less time.

As with other points of this book, opinions differ, but I advocate relatively slow movements. When you move the weight slowly, you avoid momentum effects that cause you to work the muscle less. With time under tension as a guide, the number of repetitions done is less important than the amount of time spent doing them in terms of stimulus to the muscle. But it's normally easier to count reps than to time yourself, and reps are the standard measure of work done in a set.

Some trainers advocate so-called "super slow" movements; for instance, you might take 5 seconds or longer to move the weight over your head in a shoulder press, and an equal amount of time to lower it, for a total of 10 or more seconds per rep. This can be an effective way to train for strength, but is very metabolically demanding; super-slow can also be a good method of overcoming plateaus when trying to increase strength. I lift at a slow tempo, but not "super slow".

The metabolic workout

We've discussed high-intensity training in a previous chapter, and this type of exercise provides a fine metabolic and cardiorespiratory workout. It raises heart and respiratory rates and if done regularly increases aerobic fitness and results in improved metabolic health, including better insulin sensitivity.

Strength training itself can make for a great metabolic workout. Most people who have never lifted weights may not realize the metabolic component in it. Most strength training exercises greatly increase heart and respiratory rates.

To make your strength training even more metabolic, take only short rest intervals between sets of exercise. Doing this turns your session into something more like high-intensity training, and will increase metabolic and cardiorespiratory fitness.

A bit of a compromise exists between training for strength and training for metabolic health. Generally, lighter weights, more reps, and shorter rest intervals skew the workout and give it more of a metabolic component; heavier weights, fewer reps, and longer rest intervals skew more towards strength. Bodybuilders aiming for large gains in muscle growth may use heavier weights for fewer reps and may take longer rest intervals between sets. Some of them might go to the extreme of lifting weights so heavy that they can only perform two or three reps with it. At that point, metabolic and cardiovascular elements are much less involved, and it becomes a workout for pure strength and muscle growth only. This method of strength training is for advanced practitioners.

On the other hand, using short rest intervals, lighter weights, and more reps per set and emphasizing the metabolic aspect of your workout may mean that you do not provide your muscles with the optimal growth stimulus. But for most people, there will be stimulus enough, so there's nothing to be concerned about in that regard.

Note that I'm not advocating that you work yourself to exhaustion in the gym, only that you can emphasize – or not – the metabolic aspect. By all means use fewer reps and rest up between sets if you need to.

How long is a short rest interval? At times it may be nothing at all: you just immediately move to the next exercise. At other times it could be a minute, perhaps longer, depending on your fitness level. In contrast, bodybuilders lifting heavy weights may take up to 5 minute rest intervals between sets.

Strength training for the elderly and ill

In this book, I've noted a number of studies in which elderly or ill people – for instance, people in their 90s, or with diabetes, or recovering from a hip fracture – have performed strength training programs, and how this can provide great health benefits to them. How does strength training for these groups of people differ from that for the not-so-old, and otherwise healthy people?

For one thing, they absolutely need a doctor's clearance and permission to undertake strength training, or indeed any form of exercise. In fact, everyone should have this.

Elderly and infirm people, or people with illnesses, in addition to a doctor's permission, should have solid supervision from someone who knows what he or she is doing. That person may be a physical trainer, or physical therapist, or some other experienced and knowledgeable person, who is qualified to instruct and supervise a training program. Supervision of this sort can often be found in a structured exercise program, or in exercise classes. Good instruction and supervision will ensure that the participant remains injury-free and that the exercise program is effective and does what it's supposed to do.

Fed versus fasted workouts

Some consideration should be given to what you eat around workout time, as this can be important to your results in terms of both fat loss and muscle gain.

If you want to emphasize fat loss in your strength training program, you can work out in the gym in the fasted state, meaning that you haven't eaten for at least the previous eight hours or possibly longer. This type of workout may be easier and more convenient if you normally exercise relatively early in the morning. (A cup of coffee without sugar doesn't count as breaking a fast, so you can have that in the morning before a fasted workout.) Many people have difficulty training fasted, however, and feel the need for some fuel in their bodies before hitting the gym. I've never had a problem with fasted workouts, and have worked out fasted or fed depending on my goals.

When in the fasted state, insulin levels are normally low, as they must be to burn fat. When you eat carbohydrates and protein, insulin levels rise, and depending on how high they rise, this may all but abolish the action of the cell machinery involved in fat metabolism. Training in the fasted state with the fat-burning machinery in the "on" position allows for higher levels of fat burning, as the training itself ramps up the process.

To emphasize muscle growth, you should eat within a couple of hours before your workout. Muscle growth requires the availability of the essential amino acids, and these are provided by dietary protein, which comes from meat, eggs, dairy products, and certain plant sources like nuts. The only substantial pool of amino acids in the body is in the muscle itself, so protein must be eaten either right before or right after the workout session to stimulate muscle growth. You don't want to do all that work in the gym for no results.

Many or most people who are serious about strength training and adding muscle take a protein supplement, most often whey protein. Drinking a protein shake with about 25 grams of whey protein either immediately before or after the workout provides a large amount of essential amino acids to the muscle, where they are used for muscle growth. A strength training session greatly increases the molecular muscle-growing machinery, but it then needs amino acids from protein for growth.

Whether taking protein before or after a workout provides the optimal stimulus for muscle growth has been the topic of a nearly endless debate in the strength training community, with scores of scientific papers written about it. No clear conclusions have come from it, the consensus at the moment being as long as you get some high-quality protein in the amount of 20 grams or more you'll get optimal muscle growth, and whether it's before or after a workout may make little difference.

I prefer to look at this issue from the perspective of my goals. When I want to emphasize muscle growth, I take whey protein before my workout. Whey is rapidly absorbed and its amino acids quickly reach the blood stream and the muscles, so that during the workout, as muscle-growth machinery ramps up, the muscles already have a ready supply of material with which to grow.

Recently, when I wanted to lose about 5 pounds of fat, I went back to fasted workouts and took my protein drink after my gym session. The amount of protein in whey or indeed any other type of protein is enough to raise insulin levels and to dampen fat-burning. If your goal is fat loss, save the protein for after the workout.

The best diet for strength training is a topic around which entire books have been written, and here as elsewhere there's plenty of disagreement when it comes to fine-tuning it. Generally, people new to strength training need somewhat more protein than usual, since their muscles are growing faster. In contrast, veteran bodybuilders need less protein than beginners, both because their bodies become more efficient at using protein, and because their muscles are no longer growing as fast as those of beginners.

Even veteran bodybuilders need more protein for optimal growth than non-athletes, however. How much protein is that? A number of studies have found that around 1.2 grams of protein per kilogram of body weight keeps bodybuilders in "nitrogen balance", meaning that they are neither gaining nor losing muscle mass, and that 1.8 grams of protein per kilogram of body weight is the most anyone can use for muscle growth.[103]

If you're new to strength training, want to maximize muscle, and weigh 70 kilograms (154 pounds), you therefore need at most 126 grams of protein daily. After several months to a year of training, you'll be a veteran and your protein needs will decrease to under 100 grams a day.

Good evidence also exists that dietary protein should be distributed throughout the day, i.e. not eaten at one sitting. The minimum amount of protein per meal for good muscle growth and retention is about 20 grams.

The best diet for strength training therefore should be one that contains at least 20 grams of protein, preferably animal protein, per meal. If you're a vegetarian, I strongly recommend the use of eggs and dairy products that will help you get enough protein for strength training. For the best body composition, all strength trainers should avoid highly processed foods that contain sugar or large amounts of refined carbohydrates. Emphasize whole, unprocessed foods: meat, eggs, dairy, vegetables, fruit, tubers, and nuts. (Don't even glance at the nonsense that goes under the name of the USDA food pyramid.) Some trainers and serious bodybuilders like to eat a fair amount of carbohydrates in the form of things like oatmeal or rice, and if you work hard and often in the gym, that's perfectly fine; but if you're trying to lose fat, those sources of abundant carbohydrates are best avoided. If you're thirsty, drink coffee or tea without sugar, or water, and if you drink alcohol, don't drink anything sweet.

Sample workouts

All of the above contained a lot of generalities about how to train for strength, so let's look at a couple of sample workouts.

Beginner:

Warmup
Squats: 2 sets of 8 reps each
Leg press: 1 set, 8 reps
Chest press: 2 sets at 8 reps each
Cable flies, or alternatively, dips: 2 sets
Machine shoulder press: 2 sets, 8 reps

Dumbbell shoulder press: 2 sets, 8 reps

T-bar rows: 3 sets, 8 reps

Pull-ups: 3 sets, as many reps as you can do per set

Two-way split routine

Workout A

Deadlift, 3 sets, 5 to 8 reps each

T-bar rows: 3 to 4 sets, 8 reps each

Pull-ups: 3 sets, as many reps as possible per set (you can alternate sets of rows with pull-ups)

Chest press: 3 sets, 8 to 12 reps each

Cable flies: 2 sets, 8 reps each (you can alternate sets of chest press with cable flies)

Weighted dips: 3 sets at 8 reps each with an added 45 lb plate (use less weight if needed)

Triceps pull-downs: 3 sets, 8 to 10 reps each

Biceps curls: 5 sets, 8 reps each (I like to alternate triceps pull-downs and curls)

Workout B

Squats: 3 to 4 sets, 8 reps each

Leg press: 3 sets, 8 reps each

Calf raises: 2 to 3 sets (I alternate leg press and calf-raise sets)

Machine shoulder press: 2 sets, 8 to 10 reps each

Dumbbell lateral shoulder raise: 2 sets, 8 to 10 reps (I alternate shoulder press with lateral raises)

Upright row: 3 sets, 8 reps each

Weighted chin-ups: 3 sets, 6 to 8 reps, with added 45 lb plate (or less if needed)

Barbell shoulder shrugs: 4 sets, 8 reps each

Crunches: 2 sets, as many reps as possible

Captain's chair: 2 sets, 10 to 12 reps

As with high-intensity training, the ways that a workout can be structured are nearly infinite, so these are just samples. The spit routine is close to the way I train. I haven't explained every one of these exercises in this book, because I wanted to focus on the main compound lifts and how you can get going with them, but the other exercises mentioned are easy enough to learn, and you'll see plenty of people doing them in the gym. There are many, many other exercises that you can learn if you want.

Also note the presence of a few non-compound exercises, such as shoulder shrugs and biceps curls. After you get experienced and know and can perform the main compound lifts, you can add these. There's nothing at all wrong with non-compound exercises, it's just that too many people think they'll improve their health and build muscle with only these kinds of exercises, and that is just not the case. I see many people in the gym who appear to exclusively do them; but to get strong and healthy you have to do the squats, rows, bench, etc.

As you develop more strength, add weight to your exercises. As you get more advanced, you can add more sets and expand the variety of your routine.

Questions and answers

The following are some questions, and my answers, that beginners and even experienced lifters often have about how to train.

What dietary supplements are useful in strength training?

The fitness industry sells a huge array of supplements, but which of them really work is another question entirely.

The two supplements that have the soundest scientific backing for their effectiveness are creatine and whey protein.

Creatine is a natural substance found mainly in meat, and is also synthesized in human muscle. By taking creatine as a supplement, you can boost its level in muscle. Creatine functions as an energy storage molecule, and supplementing it allows greater workout intensity and time to failure. Some studies have shown increased muscle growth with creatine too. The normal dose is about 0.03 grams per kilogram of body eight a day; so a 70-kilogram man might take around 2 grams daily. Creatine also accumulates in muscle over time – days to weeks – so it need not be taken daily. While creatine is generally considered safe, those with impaired kidney function or any other illness should consult their doctor before using it.

Whey protein, as discussed in the section on diet, has been shown to robustly increase muscle protein synthesis when taken either immediately before or after a workout. Whey is about 50% essential amino acids, contains about 25% branched-chain amino acids, and is rapidly absorbed, making it nearly the perfect muscle growth stimulator. There's also good evidence that whey can help fat loss too.

Good progress in a strength training program requires that you be well-nourished, and so supplements that conduce to good health generally are also useful for weightlifters. They include vitamin D, magnesium, and fish oil.

Many other strength training supplements exist, some with decent scientific backing for their efficacy, and some without. I use a rule of thumb: the more the supplement costs, the less effective it is.

What is the minimum effective dose of strength training?

Let's suppose that you don't like to exercise much, and you especially don't like lifting weights, but you want the health benefits. How little can you do to get those benefits?

Anything at all, no matter how minimal, will have some effect. But if you want to see gains in strength and better body composition, you could do this in a once weekly training session, provided this workout is intense enough. If you were doing the one set to failure method, and did the five main compound exercises, you could be out of the gym in under 30 minutes. Be sure to be physically active on most other days also.

You won't become the next Arnold Schwarzenegger doing this, but you should see solid improvements in health and strength.

Can I work out daily?

Some people don't have any problem with daily workouts, but I'm certainly not one of them and don't recommend them. If your workouts are intense enough, as they should be, your muscles and your entire body need rest, since muscles grow when they're resting, not in the gym.

If you perform whole-body workouts, I recommend a minimum of one rest day between sessions. Some people may need more, especially if some other, non-strength exercise is done on off-days. Split workouts are a different story, since we're not training the same muscle group daily. In a 4-way split workout, you could conceivably train as much as four times a week.

In daily strength training, you run the risk of applying too much stress to your body and causing it to be in a constant state of breakdown, possibly leading to worse health. I know some guys who are in the gym almost daily, and one thing I often hear from them is that they don't feel very energetic, that they're listless and not up for a hard workout; but they never get the connection between the lack of proper rest and feeling unwell. Don't do this. Apply the appropriate and optimal stimulus for strength gains, but also realize that in weightlifting, less is often more.

Do you need a basal level of strength before you start?

In theory it's certainly possible that someone could be too weak or debilitated to take up strength training, but as we've seen in this book, even quite old and weak people have benefited from some form of it. In practice, most people can start to train just by using lighter weights, even 2-pound dumbbells, and easing into it. Body weight exercises—push-ups, air squats, and the like – may be a good place to start if you feel that you're too weak to train with weights. Certain categories of people, such as the old and/or ill, need a doctor's clearance and a supervised exercise program.

What's the deal with abs?

Having prominent abdominal muscles – abs – has come to be seen as a requirement for a truly great body, mainly in men. The reality is that they can be fairly hard to get, which is of course one reason they're seen as so desirable.

Building abs as a muscle is not difficult: sit-ups and crunches, whether weighted or not, easily build the abs. The "secret" to abs lies in making them visible, and the only thing that will do this is a low body fat percentage. Everyone has abs, they merely need to be uncovered. If you want ripped abs, your goal should be fat loss.

But it should be said that much of the demand for ripped abs is a media creation, designed to sell magazines and books. Not many people really have them, and they're not necessary to be in excellent health and fine shape. Getting them takes a lot of work and discipline, so if you want them, be prepared.

Should I use heavier weights or more reps for better gains in strength and health?

There's a spectrum of health effects associated with strength training, with pure strength on one end of the spectrum, and cardiometabolic fitness on the other. Generally, with lighter weights and more reps, you move toward the cardiorespiratory and metabolic fitness end of the spectrum; with heavier weights and fewer reps, you move toward the muscle strength end of the spectrum. The rep range of 8 to 12 appears to be optimal for stimulating muscle growth.

But even this has been challenged. Recent research has found that, as long as you lift to failure, lighter weights can provide as much or even more stimulus for muscle growth as heavier weights.[104] This occurs because with more reps in the set, you actually end up doing more work, defined as weight x repetitions.

Lifting heavier weights also makes injury more likely than lifting lighter. If you lift heavy weights, respect their power and make sure you can handle them to stay injury-free.

Do I risk injury to joints over the long term?

Strength training, as we saw above, has a lower rate of injuries than distance running. If strength training moves are done with good form, they align with the joints' natural movement, and the number of reps in any move is not high, avoiding excessive wear and tear. By contrast, running involves stress on hips, ankles, and feet, repeated thousands of times in just one bout of exercise, leading to overuse and lots of wear and tear. Strength training appears to have a low potential for joint injuries.

Tendons may be more susceptible to injury, as they need to become stronger as well and may take longer to do so than muscles. Here again, good form is the best way to prevent injury.

How do I get motivated to do my workout?

Good question. I personally don't have much trouble getting motivated for any kind of exercise. My motivation comes from knowing that I'm improving my health and seeing beneficial changes in body composition, and I want those to continue. Exercise also improves my mood, so that's a great motivator – I can look forward to having a brighter outlook on life after my workout. When you start to see that your health and body comp are improving, and notice how a workout affects your mood, hopefully that will be sufficient motivation to get you into the gym.

Coffee works too. Seriously, I won't go to the gym without some caffeine. Coffee also helps burn fat and has an analgesic effect, which is why they put it in headache pills. All of those effects will get you through your workout a bit easier.

Lots of people in the gym have done way better than me. What gives?

Assuming that you work out as hard as others, and eat and sleep as well as others, there is one factor over which you have no control: your genes.

It's been said that the most important step in becoming an Olympic athlete is choosing the right parents. Genes are just that important to athletic ability, and that includes the ability to grow muscles and lose fat.

Genes control and set limits to the levels of hormones such as growth hormone, IGF-1, myostatin, and testosterone, all of them important to strength training. Genes set limits to VO_2max, hemoglobin levels, and even your enthusiasm for exercise. There is a large genetic component to every aspect of physiology and behavior. In some cases the genetic component may approach 100%, making it difficult to overcome – your height, for example. A small number of people hardly even respond to exercise due to their genes. In other cases the genetic component is smaller, and hard work can mitigate it – your body fat percentage, for example.

It's difficult to know when your training has bumped up against genetic limits. In the first year of strength training, many beginners can easily gain 30 or more pounds of muscle, and I did that myself. After the first year, adding muscle becomes a lot harder, and after several years, one shouldn't expect more than a few pounds of muscle gain annually. You've reached your genetic potential as far as muscle growth, or have come very close to it.

Same goes for fat loss and body fat percentage. While after a few months of training some people will become nearly "shredded" (very low body fat), others will have difficulty losing as much fat as they would like.

None of this is a counsel of despair, because the environment, including exercise, diet, sleep, and so on, is still under your control. Concentrate on what you can change, not what you can't.

One clue as to your genetics comes from family members: if they tend to be on the stocky side, for instance, you will probably add muscle more readily and perhaps have more difficulty in losing fat than if your family tends to the thin side. My father allegedly weighed 125 pounds at 6 feet tall at age 22, but that didn't stop me from adding lots of muscle through strength training, so don't let an alleged genetic component stop you from giving it your all.

Should I have other types of exercise in my rotation besides strength training?

Not necessarily. If you train for strength with intensity and more than once a week, that may be close to all you need not just for strength, but for good metabolic and cardiorespiratory health.

However, there's a difference between not exercising intensely on non-training days, and being completely sedentary. Being sedentary is associated with much worse health, and this applies even if you regularly exercise. Sitting for long periods of time, more than four hours daily, is associated with worse insulin sensitivity, greater obesity, and higher cardiovascular and all-cause mortality.[105]

So, while you don't necessarily need to do any intense or hard exercise other than strength training, don't be a couch potato when outside the gym. Walking is a great exercise that keeps you from being sedentary yet is not so intense that it impairs your recovery time from strength training. I try to walk for at least a couple of miles on every off-gym day.

If you have a job in which you must sit at a desk for hours at a time, take frequent breaks and get up, stretch, move around, maybe walk around the block if feasible. Or eat lunch at your desk and walk on your lunch break.

High-intensity training sessions may be added to your routine if you want to do relatively intense exercise on days when you are not training for strength. But don't overdo it, and be aware of your body and whether it needs more rest. If it does, just go for a walk.

Should I change the way I lift, such as type of exercise, reps, weight, and frequency, as I get older?

Age affects energy levels, ability to recover from exercise, tendency to get injured, and many other things. But different people are affected by age differently. There are some people in their 70s or older who are in better shape and can out-lift much younger people.

Age by itself is no reason to change the way you train: the same principles of strength training apply to all ages. But you must be aware of what you are capable of. If a tendon aches after a set or session, you will need to adjust your routine around it. If you have a back problem, then maybe deadlifts are not for you. If your recovery time is higher, then you need more rest days between sessions. However, these caveats apply whether you are 30 or 80.

If you are older, or as you become older, you merely need to be cognizant of your body's capabilities.

How can I get big and strong, fast?

When it comes to building muscle, there's no substitute for hard work. If you want to get big, do multiple sets at high intensity. for example, use a weight heavy enough that you can do only 8 reps with it, rest several minutes between sets, and do up to 8 sets. Do a split workout such that you exercise each muscle group at high volume once a week. For instance, you might have a dedicated leg day, when you do only squats and leg presses, a dedicated chest day, etc.

You're going to have to be dedicated to do this, because you're going to need lots of recovery time and lots of sleep.

The other factor is nutrition: make sure you get plenty of calories and protein, up to 1.8 grams of protein per kilogram of body weight daily. Doing this will likely require protein supplementation with whey or casein, perhaps up to 50 grams daily, which would mean a twice daily protein shake.

Calories are another matter, because you can end up putting on a lot of body fat, so don't go overboard. I don't believe in bulking, the practice of forcing yourself to eat a lot in order to gain weight. Certainly, if you want to get big, don't let yourself get hungry very often, but don't force feed yourself either. Calorie consumption needs to be matched more or less with your progress in the gym in order to gain more muscle than fat. If you bulk and end up putting on more fat than muscle, it can be very hard to lose, and you can harm your metabolism by increasing insulin resistance.

Afterword

Exercise greatly improves health, and hardly anything else even comes close to its power. Other lifestyle factors, such as diet and sleep, are also important, but for many people the single best thing they could do for their health is to start exercising.

Exercise works by acting as a stress which signals the body to increase its physiological stress defense mechanisms and its capacity to perform at a high level. In this way, the immune system, cardiorespiratory fitness, insulin sensitivity and other aspects of metabolic health, detoxifying enzymes, and other systems all improve in function.

The intensity of exercise must rise above a certain threshold before it causes beneficial effects. This threshold depends not only on the type, intensity, and duration of exercise, but on the person doing the exercise. Walking, for instance, will improve the fitness of a sedentary person, but will do little to nothing for a person accustomed to running long distances. Air squats may be a tremendous workout for an older person used to sitting in a chair all the time, but won't do much for an experienced bodybuilder.

The type of exercise almost universally recommended by mainstream health authorities over the past several decades has been steady-state aerobic exercise. In order for this type of exercise to be effective at improving health, it substitutes duration for intensity. Aerobic exercise is usually performed at such an intensity that it can be kept up for quite awhile, in some cases for hours, as in distance running. Even the lower level sort of aerobics, such as running on a treadmill or using an elliptical machine, are designed so that the user exercises for 10, 20, 30 minutes at a stretch, or even longer.

Exercise of higher intensity, such as strength training or high-intensity interval training (HIT), consist of short bouts of higher intensity than aerobics, lasting at most a few minutes a bout, and done in a sequence. Yet strength training and HIT have demonstrated as great a capacity for increasing cardiorespiratory and metabolic fitness as aerobic exercise, or even more so.

From these considerations it can be seen that aerobic exercise is inefficient and unnecessary for fitness. The idea behind aerobic exercise is that it has a unique ability, through a combination of its low level and duration, to increase fitness. But it does not: increase the intensity of the exercise and the length of time necessary for the exercise to improve fitness drops dramatically.

Because of its relatively long duration, aerobic exercise also has a higher rate of injuries, which mainly occurs through overuse.

Another consequence of the perception that aerobic exercise is the only one that matters is that the most common excuse people use for not exercising is lack of time. Rightly or wrongly, many people feel that they don't have many hours a week to devote to exercise.

Aerobic exercise also has little ability to aid fat loss or to stave off the increasing muscle loss of aging. It may even accelerate muscle loss in some cases.

In contrast to aerobics, strength training has been the poor stepchild of exercise, recommended by hardly anyone and seen generally as the province of muscle-obsessed bodybuilders. Fortunately, this is beginning to change, as doctors and others in health care understand its great benefits.

In this book, I've shown the reader why he or she should add strength training and/or high-intensity interval training to his or her exercise program, and even why they can be the main or even only elements of that program. Far from being the exclusive province of bodybuilders, it can improve the health of almost anyone, by helping fat loss, muscle gain, and preventing cancer and heart disease. It can prevent many older people from a life of dependence, frailty, and institutional living, and can help everyone to be fit and have an attractive body.

About the author

P. D. Mangan is the author of four previous books on health and fitness: **Smash Chronic Fatigue**; **Best Supplements for Men's Health, Strength, and Virility**; **Top Ten Reasons We're Fat**; and **Stop the Clock: The Optimal Anti-Aging Strategy**; all are available at Amazon.

Sign up for newsletter updates at my website, **Rogue Health and Fitness**, and get my guide to intermittent fasting.

If you enjoyed this book, I'd appreciate it if you'd consider leaving a review on the book's Amazon page. And tell your friends!

1   http://suewidemark.com/fat-fit-new.htm

2   Mekary, Rania A., et al. "Weight training, aerobic physical activities, and long-term waist circumference change in men." Obesity 23.2 (2015): 461-467.

3   Lean-washing: Profiting from misinformation on what causes obesity http://ns.umich.edu/new/releases/22264-lean-washing-profiting-from-misinformation-on-what-causes-obesity

4   Malhotra, A., T. Noakes, and S. Phinney. "It is time to bust the myth of physical inactivity and obesity: you cannot outrun a bad diet." British journal of sports medicine (2015): bjsports-2015.

5   Siegel, Rebecca L., Kimberly D. Miller, and Ahmedin Jemal. "Cancer statistics, 2015." CA: a cancer journal for clinicians 65.1 (2015): 5-29.

6   http://www.cancer.gov/about-cancer/causes-prevention/risk/obesity/obesity-fact-sheet

7   Calle, Eugenia E., et al. "Overweight, obesity, and mortality from cancer in a prospectively studied cohort of US adults." New England Journal of Medicine 348.17 (2003): 1625-1638.

8   http://www.cancer.org/cancer/cancercauses/dietandphysicalactivity/bodyweightandcancerrisk/body-weight-and-cancer-risk-effects

9   Kampert, James B., et al. "Physical activity, physical fitness, and all-cause and cancer mortality: a prospective study of men and women." Annals of epidemiology 6.5 (1996): 452-457.

10 Ruiz, Jonatan R., et al. "Muscular strength and adiposity as predictors of adulthood cancer mortality in men." Cancer Epidemiology Biomarkers & Prevention 18.5 (2009): 1468-1476.

11 Izquierdo, Mikel, et al. "Differential effects of strength training leading to failure versus not to failure on hormonal responses, strength, and muscle power gains." Journal of Applied Physiology 100.5 (2006): 1647-1656.

12 Steuerman, Rachel, Orit Shevah, and Zvi Laron. "Congenital IGF1

deficiency tends to confer protection against post-natal development of malignancies." European Journal of Endocrinology 164.4 (2011): 485-489.

13 Yu, Herbert, and Thomas Rohan. "Role of the insulin-like growth factor family in cancer development and progression." Journal of the National Cancer Institute 92.18 (2000): 1472-1489.

14 Walker, KYLIE S., et al. "Resistance training alters plasma myostatin but not IGF-1 in healthy men." Medicine and science in sports and exercise 36.5 (2004): 787-793.

15 Kaaks, Rudulf. "Nutrition, hormones, and breast cancer: is insulin the missing link?." Cancer Causes & Control 7.6 (1996): 605-625.

16 Giovannucci, E. "Modifiable risk factors for colon cancer." Gastroenterology clinics of North America 31.4 (2002): 925-943.

17 Khandwala, Hasnain M., et al. "The effects of insulin-like growth factors on tumorigenesis and neoplastic growth." Endocrine reviews 21.3 (2000): 215-244.

18 Ishii, Tomofusa, et al. "Resistance training improves insulin sensitivity in NIDDM subjects without altering maximal oxygen uptake." Diabetes care 21.8 (1998): 1353-1355.

19 Dela, Flemming, and Michael Kjaer. "Resistance training, insulin sensitivity and muscle function in the elderly." Essays Biochem 42 (2006): 75-88.

20 Holten, Mads K., et al. "Strength training increases insulin-mediated glucose uptake, GLUT4 content, and insulin signaling in skeletal muscle in patients with type 2 diabetes." Diabetes 53.2 (2004): 294-305.

21 Pedersen, Bente Klarlund, et al. "Role of myokines in exercise and metabolism." Journal of applied physiology 103.3 (2007): 1093-1098.

22 Gannon, Nicholas P., et al. "Effects of the exercise-inducible myokine irisin on malignant and non-malignant breast epithelial cell behavior in vitro." International Journal of Cancer 136.4 (2015): E197-E202.

23 Hardee, Justin P., et al. "The effect of resistance exercise on all-cause mortality in cancer survivors." Mayo Clinic Proceedings. Vol. 89. No. 8. Elsevier, 2014.

24 Thijs, Karin M., et al. "Rehabilitation using high-intensity physical training and long-term return-to-work in cancer survivors." Journal of occupational rehabilitation 22.2 (2012): 220-229.

25 Giovannucci, Edward L. "Physical activity as a standard cancer treatment." Journal of the National Cancer Institute 104.11 (2012): 797-799.

26 Gallot, Yann S., et al. "Myostatin Gene Inactivation Prevents Skeletal Muscle Wasting in Cancer." Cancer research 74.24 (2014): 7344-7356.

27 Marcora, Samuele M., Andrew B. Lemmey, and Peter J. Maddison. "Can progressive resistance training reverse cachexia in patients with rheumatoid arthritis? Results of a pilot study." The Journal of rheumatology 32.6 (2005): 1031-1039.

28 Ruas, Jorge L., et al. "A PGC-1α isoform induced by resistance training regulates skeletal muscle hypertrophy." Cell 151.6 (2012): 1319-1331.

29 Strasser, Barbara, et al. "Impact of resistance training in cancer survivors: a meta-analysis." Med Sci Sports Exerc 45.11 (2013): 2080-2090.

30 Mendias, Christopher L., et al. "Haploinsufficiency of myostatin protects against aging-related declines in muscle function and enhances the longevity of mice." Aging cell (2015).

31 Walker, KYLIE S., et al. "Resistance training alters plasma myostatin but not IGF-1 in healthy men." Medicine and science in sports and exercise 36.5 (2004): 787-793.

32 http://www.cdc.gov/heartdisease/facts.htm

33 http://www.strokeassociation.org/STROKEORG/AboutStroke/Impact-of-Stroke-Stroke-statistics_UCM_310728_Article.jsp

34 Sasaki, Hideo, et al. "Grip strength predicts cause-specific mortality in middle-aged and elderly persons." The American journal of medicine

120.4 (2007): 337-342.

35   Gale, Catharine R., et al. "Grip strength, body composition, and mortality."
     International journal of epidemiology 36.1 (2007): 228-235.

36   Cornelissen, Véronique A., et al. "Impact of resistance training on blood
     pressure and other cardiovascular risk factors a meta-analysis of
     randomized, controlled trials." Hypertension 58.5 (2011): 950-958.

37   Braith, Randy W., and Kerry J. Stewart. "Resistance exercise training its
     role in the prevention of cardiovascular disease." Circulation 113.22
     (2006): 2642-2650.

38   Ruiz, Jonatan R., et al. "Association between muscular strength and
     mortality in men: prospective cohort study." Bmj 337 (2008): a439.

39   Ozaki, Hayao, et al. "Resistance training induced increase in VO2max in
     young and older subjects." European Review of Aging and Physical
     Activity 10.2 (2013): 107-116.

40   Hagerman, Fredrick C., et al. "Effects of high-intensity resistance training
     on untrained older men. I. Strength, cardiovascular, and metabolic
     responses." The journals of gerontology series A: Biological Sciences and
     medical sciences 55.7 (2000): B336-B346.

41   Vincent, Kevin R., et al. "Improved cardiorespiratory endurance following
     6 months of resistance exercise in elderly men and women." Archives of
     Internal Medicine 162.6 (2002): 673-678.

42   Williams, Mark A., et al. "Resistance exercise in individuals with and
     without cardiovascular disease: 2007 update a scientific statement from the
     american heart association council on clinical cardiology and council on
     nutrition, physical activity, and metabolism." Circulation 116.5 (2007):
     572-584.

43   http://eatingacademy.com/why-i-decided-to-lose-weight

44   Wolfe, Robert R. "The underappreciated role of muscle in health and
     disease." The American journal of clinical nutrition 84.3 (2006): 475-482.

45 Bryner, Randy W., et al. "Effects of resistance vs. aerobic training combined with an 800 calorie liquid diet on lean body mass and resting metabolic rate." Journal of the American College of Nutrition 18.2 (1999): 115-121.

46 Demling, Robert H., and Leslie DeSanti. "Effect of a hypocaloric diet, increased protein intake and resistance training on lean mass gains and fat mass loss in overweight police officers." Annals of Nutrition and Metabolism 44.1 (2000): 21-29.

47 Mekary, Rania A., et al. "Weight training, aerobic physical activities, and long-term waist circumference change in men." Obesity 23.2 (2015): 461-467.

48 Romero-Corral, Abel, et al. "Normal weight obesity: a risk factor for cardiometabolic dysregulation and cardiovascular mortality." European Heart Journal (2009): ehp487.

49 Jackson, Allen W., et al. "Muscular strength is inversely related to prevalence and incidence of obesity in adult men." Obesity 18.10 (2010): 1988-1995.

50 Berentzen, Tina Landsvig, et al. "Changes in waist circumference and mortality in middle-aged men and women." PLoS One 5.9 (2010): e13097.

51 Westcott, Wayne L., et al. "Prescribing physical activity: applying the ACSM protocols for exercise type, intensity, and duration across 3 training frequencies." The Physician and sportsmedicine 37.2 (2009): 51-58.

52 Hackney, A. C. "Effects of endurance exercise on the reproductive system of men: the "exercise-hypogonadal male condition"." Journal of endocrinological investigation 31.10 (2008): 932-938.

53 Faulkner, John A., et al. "Age-related changes in the structure and function of skeletal muscles." Clinical and Experimental Pharmacology and Physiology 34.11 (2007): 1091-1096.

54 LeBlanc, Erin S., et al. "Hip fracture and increased short-term but not long-term mortality in healthy older women." Archives of internal medicine 171.20 (2011): 1831-1837.

55 Evans, William J. "Skeletal muscle loss: cachexia, sarcopenia, and inactivity." The American journal of clinical nutrition 91.4 (2010): 1123S-1127S.

56 Evans, William J. "Skeletal muscle loss: cachexia, sarcopenia, and inactivity." The American journal of clinical nutrition 91.4 (2010): 1123S-1127S.

57 McWhirter, Janet P., and Christopher R. Pennington. "Incidence and recognition of malnutrition in hospital." Bmj 308.6934 (1994): 945-948.

58 Pereira, C. T., et al. "Age-dependent differences in survival after severe burns: a unicentric review of 1,674 patients and 179 autopsies over 15 years." Journal of the American College of Surgeons 202.3 (2006): 536.

59 Layne, JENNIFER E., and MIRIAM E. Nelson. "The effects of progressive resistance training on bone density: a review." Medicine and science in sports and exercise 31.1 (1999): 25-30.

60 Frost, Harold M. "On our age-related bone loss: insights from a new paradigm." Journal of Bone and Mineral Research 12.10 (1997): 1539-1546.

61 Watson, S. L., et al. "Heavy resistance training is safe and improves bone, function, and stature in postmenopausal women with low to very low bone mass: novel early findings from the LIFTMOR trial." Osteoporosis International (2015): 1-6.

62 Baylis, Daniel, et al. "Understanding how we age: insights into inflammaging." Longev Healthspan 2.1 (2013): 8.

63 Rennie, M. J., et al. "Facts, noise and wishful thinking: muscle protein turnover in aging and human disuse atrophy." Scandinavian journal of medicine & science in sports 20.1 (2010): 5-9.

64 Frank, P., et al. "Strength training improves muscle aerobic capacity and glucose tolerance in elderly." Scandinavian journal of medicine & science in sports (2015).

65 Dunstan, David W., et al. "High-intensity resistance training improves

glycemic control in older patients with type 2 diabetes." Diabetes care 25.10 (2002): 1729-1736.

66 Hurley, Ben F., and Stephen M. Roth. "Strength training in the elderly." Sports Medicine 30.4 (2000): 249-268.

67 Singh, Nalin A., et al. "Effects of high-intensity progressive resistance training and targeted multidisciplinary treatment of frailty on mortality and nursing home admissions after hip fracture: a randomized controlled trial." Journal of the American Medical Directors Association 13.1 (2012): 24-30.

68 http://www.cdc.gov/homeandrecreationalsafety/falls/adultfalls.html

69 http://www.medicareadvocacy.org/old-site/News/Archives/RehabHosp_RehabOptions.htm

70 Yarrow, Joshua F., et al. "Training augments resistance exercise induced elevation of circulating brain derived neurotrophic factor (BDNF)." Neuroscience letters 479.2 (2010): 161-165.

71 Nagamatsu, Lindsay S., et al. "Resistance training promotes cognitive and functional brain plasticity in seniors with probable mild cognitive impairment." Archives of internal medicine 172.8 (2012): 666-668.

72 Podewils, Laura Jean, et al. "Physical activity, APOE genotype, and dementia risk: findings from the Cardiovascular Health Cognition Study." American journal of epidemiology 161.7 (2005): 639-651.

73 Farmer, J., et al. "Effects of voluntary exercise on synaptic plasticity and gene expression in the dentate gyrus of adult male Sprague–Dawley rats in vivo." Neuroscience 124.1 (2004): 71-79.

74 Harman, S. Mitchell, et al. "Longitudinal effects of aging on serum total and free testosterone levels in healthy men." The Journal of Clinical Endocrinology & Metabolism 86.2 (2001): 724-731.

75 Travison, Thomas G., et al. "A population-level decline in serum testosterone levels in American men." The Journal of Clinical Endocrinology & Metabolism 92.1 (2007): 196-202.

76 Andersson, Anna-Maria, et al. "Secular decline in male testosterone and sex hormone binding globulin serum levels in Danish population surveys." The Journal of Clinical Endocrinology & Metabolism 92.12 (2007): 4696-4705.

77 Kraemer, William J., et al. "Effects of heavy-resistance training on hormonal response patterns in younger vs. older men." Journal of Applied Physiology 87.3 (1999): 982-992.

78 Wang, Christina, et al. "Low testosterone associated with obesity and the metabolic syndrome contributes to sexual dysfunction and cardiovascular disease risk in men with type 2 diabetes." Diabetes care 34.7 (2011): 1669-1675.

79 Yuki, Atsumu, et al. "Relationship between low free testosterone levels and loss of muscle mass." Scientific reports 3 (2013).

80 Sinha, Indranil, et al. "Testosterone is essential for skeletal muscle growth in aged mice in a heterochronic parabiosis model." Cell and tissue research 357.3 (2014): 815-821.

81 Hackney, A. C. "Effects of endurance exercise on the reproductive system of men: the "exercise-hypogonadal male condition"." Journal of endocrinological investigation 31.10 (2008): 932-938.

82 Maimoun, L., et al. "Testosterone is significantly reduced in endurance athletes without impact on bone mineral density." Hormone Research in Paediatrics 59.6 (2003): 285-292.

83 http://www.oldtimestrongman.com/strength-articles/iron-henry-rollins

84 Furnham, Adrian, Tina Tan, and Chris McManus. "Waist-to-hip ratio and preferences for body shape: A replication and extension." Personality and Individual Differences 22.4 (1997): 539-549.

85 Behm, David G., et al. "Canadian Society for Exercise Physiology position paper: resistance training in children and adolescents." Applied physiology, nutrition, and metabolism 33.3 (2008): 547-561.

86 Singh, Devendra. "Adaptive significance of female physical attractiveness: role of waist-to-hip ratio." Journal of personality and social psychology 65.2 (1993): 293.

87 van Gent, Bobbie RN, et al. "Incidence and determinants of lower extremity running injuries in long distance runners: a systematic review." British journal of sports medicine (2007).

88 http://well.blogs.nytimes.com/2015/05/05/treadmill-may-be-riskiest-machine-but-injuries-from-it-still-rare/

89 http://www.pedbikeinfo.org/data/factsheet_crash.cfm

90 Schnohr, Peter, et al. "Dose of jogging and long-term mortality: the Copenhagen City Heart Study." Journal of the American College of Cardiology 65.5 (2015): 411-419.

91 Breuckmann, Frank, et al. "Myocardial Late Gadolinium Enhancement: Prevalence, Pattern, and Prognostic Relevance in Marathon Runners1." Radiology (2009).

92 Wilson, Mathew, et al. "Diverse patterns of myocardial fibrosis in lifelong, veteran endurance athletes." Journal of Applied Physiology 110.6 (2011): 1622-1626.

93 http://www.strengthandconditioningresearch.com/2014/07/08/injury-strength-sports/

94 Gibala, Martin J., et al. "Physiological adaptations to low-volume, high-intensity interval training in health and disease." The Journal of physiology 590.5 (2012): 1077-1084.

95 Tabata, Izumi, et al. "Effects of moderate-intensity endurance and high-intensity intermittent training on anaerobic capacity and VO2max." Medicine and science in sports and exercise 28.10 (1996): 1327-1330.

96 Boutcher, Stephen H. "High-intensity intermittent exercise and fat loss." Journal of obesity 2011 (2010).

97 Trapp, E. G., et al. "The effects of high-intensity intermittent exercise training on fat loss and fasting insulin levels of young women." International journal of obesity 32.4 (2008): 684-691.

98 Cassidy, Sophie, et al. "High intensity intermittent exercise improves cardiac structure and function and reduces liver fat in patients with type 2 diabetes: a randomised controlled trial." Diabetologia (2015): 1-11.

99 Emberts, Talisa, et al. "Exercise intensity and energy expenditure of a Tabata workout." Journal of sports science & medicine 12.3 (2013): 612.

100 Gliemann, Lasse, et al. "10-20-30 training increases performance and lowers blood pressure and VEGF in runners." Scandinavian journal of medicine & science in sports (2015).

101 http://www.builtlean.com/2010/08/03/ideal-body-fat-percentage-chart/

102 http://www.strengthandconditioningresearch.com/2014/07/08/injury-strength-sports/

103 http://bayesianbodybuilding.com/the-myth-of-1glb-optimal-protein-intake-for-bodybuilders/

104 Burd, Nicholas A., et al. "Low-load high volume resistance exercise stimulates muscle protein synthesis more than high-load low volume resistance exercise in young men." PloS one 5.8 (2010): e12033.

105 Owen, Neville, et al. "Too much sitting: the population-health science of sedentary behavior." Exercise and sport sciences reviews 38.3 (2010): 105.

Made in the USA
San Bernardino, CA
23 September 2018